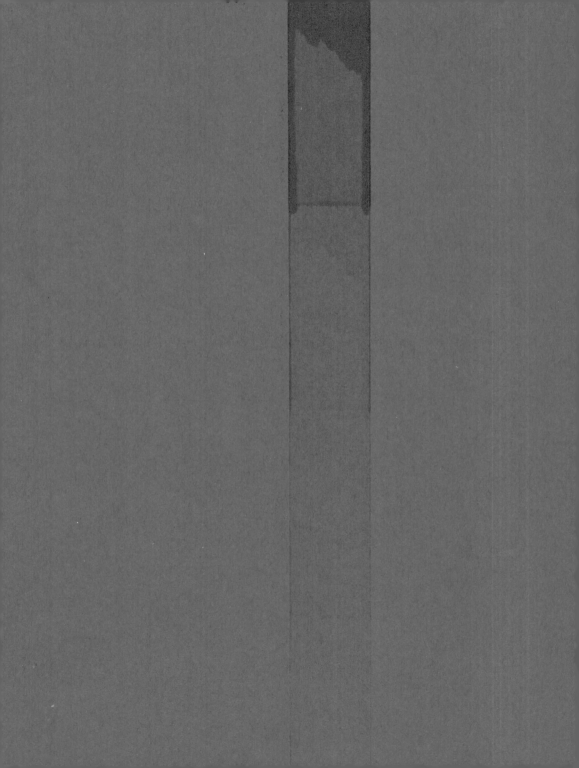

THE MAGIC KEY TO

- CHARM -

EILEEN ASCROFT

THE MAGIC KEY TO

CHARM

&

Instructions for a Delightful Life

WITH AN INTRODUCTION BY
Joanna Lumley

VINTAGE BOOKS
London

Published by Vintage 2007

2 4 6 8 10 9 7 5 3 1

Copyright © Mirrorpix 1938

Introduction copyright © Joanna Lumley 2007

The right of Eileen Ascroft to be identified as the author of this
work has been asserted under the Copyright, Designs and
Patents Act 1988

First published in Great Britain in 1938 by Hurst and Blackett, Ltd.

Random House, 20 Vauxhall Bridge Road,
London SW1V 2SA

www.vintage-books.co.uk

Addresses for companies within The Random House Group Limited
can be found at: www.randomhouse.co.uk/offices.htm

The Random House Group Limited Reg. No. 954009

A CIP catalogue record for this book is available from the British Library

ISBN 9780099518235

The Random House Group Limited makes every effort to ensure
that the papers used in its books are made from trees that have
been legally sourced from well-managed and credibly certified forests.
Our paper procurement policy can be found at:
www.randomhouse.co.uk/paper.htm

Printed and bound in Germany by
GGP Media GmbH, Pößneck

FOREWORD

Every woman wants to get the best from life and make the most of her opportunities, appearance and abilities.

I believe that Charm is the magic key to happiness and success.

And I believe that every woman has the seeds of Charm within her. She has only to learn to liberate it.

When my Charm lessons first appeared in the *Daily Mirror* there were many requests for them in a more permanent form.

This book is the result. I hope it will help you and bring you success and happiness.

Eileen Ascroft

CONTENTS

CONTENTS

INTRODUCTION

In 1964 Lucie Clayton of New Bond Street offered two courses for young women: Modelling and Charm. Modelling, which I took, involved learning two kinds of make-up, street and evening (both applied rather more lightly than the newly swinging sixties recommended); walking very smoothly with your hip-bones travelling ahead of your torso; and turning like a viper on the spot, having first crossed your legs and altered your weight so in one move you could perform a volte-face and start off back down the imaginary catwalk.

The Charm students were upstairs, I think; our paths didn't cross, as they were learning how to appreciate paintings, arrange flowers and lay a table for a dinner party. I may have partly imagined this: maybe, like us, they also learned how to get in and out of an E-type Jaguar charmingly without showing their pants. Perhaps they were being groomed to marry husbands rich enough to give them the kind of life which could involve giving dinner parties and having a guest bedroom, whereas we were headed towards the slightly murkier but more exciting avenue of hair-pieces, body stockings and false fingernails. Did we envy each other? No, not really. I should have liked to spend time in art galleries but at home I had already learned how to lay a table and serve vegetables from the left. I knew by then how to introduce Mr X to Mrs Y, that gloves and hankies should be spotless (mine weren't) and that guests and fish stink after three days. Kipling's *The Second Jungle Book* had taught me to 'Wash daily from nose-tip to tail-tip. Drink deeply but never too deep.' I had gathered, roughly, how to arrange flowers and sew on buttons: my finishing school had been my home, leaving, it must be said, much room for improvement.

So the Charm course was in effect a finishing school, a concept which even then was in danger of appearing hopelessly outmoded. Who, in those heady days of free love and happenings, wanted to wave their husband off in a clean apron and a dab of scent at the wrist? Who indeed wanted to please a MAN? The world's great see-saw was tilting and all the womanly qualities that had been admired before became risible as girls stripped off their self-effacement in the race to become more equal to men: equal in pay, freedom, jobs and behaviour. Men slept around: why couldn't girls? Men could get drunk, go out in gangs, spend their money the way they wanted: why should women slog away at home, chastely polishing and cooking, putting out the slippers and supervising homework? A seismic change began to take place which affected everyone. After the upheavals of two world wars, society had to rewrite its rules yet again, and while many of the alterations were fair and necessary, many were unhelpful and destructive. There were casualties and triumphs in equal measure: but the first thing that seemed to have been slung far out of the pram was charm. It rolled away into the bushes where it has lain under dead leaves for decades. Until now. Charm has been picked up with cries of affectionate nostalgia, dusted down and put back into the pram of the furious baby, who is now almost grown-up and has started to tire of the excesses so valued during the Me-generation.

This book, written just before the Second World War, would have resonated with women from all walks of life. To be thought of as ladylike was a common goal; elegance and modesty were attributes to be admired. Eileen Ascroft's charm lessons were printed first singly on the women's page of the *Daily Mirror*, then assembled in an album that a young woman could put on the shelf beside her Mrs Beeton (and, presumably, next to the fairly hefty reading library recommended on page 72: hard to think of a list this long appearing in any popular newspapers today). People keen to better themselves prized virtues like daintiness and humility but Miss Ascroft wanted even more than that for her pupils. She wanted them, us, to learn how to reveal the charm that she believed everyone has inside already: to grasp the Magic Key to happiness, friendship and love.

'Every woman who is worthy of the name of woman has pondered how she could bring into the world more radiance, more glamour.' As we settle back on our scuffed heels, wondering if we are worthy enough to read on, she urges: 'Do not be surprised and do not make a mistake; I am not going to teach you tricks – I know none.' What follows, chapter by chapter, is a self-help manual, advice written long ago but recycled to this day in the columns of agony aunts and reality television programmes in which demoralised lank-haired women are encouraged to shape up and take pride in their appearance.

Miss Ascroft is a thrilling advisor; like a good headmistress she expects the best from us from the start. ('You have become my pupil today . . . make a note of its date in your personal diary, because today will begin to change your life.') There are some searching questionnaires (probably pronounced 'kestionnaires') with a rap over the knuckles for achieving the lowest marks: and quite right too, as they reveal that you 'are selfish and far too self-centred' or that 'you're giving your poor husband a very bad deal'. Children don't feature much in this book, except that they should be borne without complaint: 'Some women make their husbands' lives hell by their whinings and ailments and incessant talk about the baby'. She notes crisply that the baby should fit into your household and not be a nuisance. But this isn't a book for mothers: it's for young girls, away from home for the first time, unsure of how to meet people, how to make the best of themselves, how to . . . well, how to BE, for goodness sake.

Finding which of the seven glandular theme types you are is a bit of a tooth-sucking moment. Am I the 'Man's Girl', the 'Perfect Wife' or the 'Glamorous Type'? Certainly not the 'Childishly Appealing Type', who will 'appear almost boneless'. Do I look like the sort of person I should like to meet myself? And as an older woman with grey/white hair (which has been dyed yellow) which colour scheme is suitable in a north-east-facing room? Grey and pink or the more youthful yellow and turquoise-blue? (Oh! I have just looked and by some weird coincidence our drawing room *is* golden yellow with some turquoise blue. Spot on, Miss Ascroft). But am I affected, or irritating? Do I pick at things with my fingers, hum nervously under my breath and snap my suspenders? Do I look ugly as I run for the bus, frowning clutching my bag and wobbling 'in the most ungainly way'? Have I tried to be charming to every single person I have met today?

But notice how this charm advice is going deeper, like taking the plunge with your arms around a dolphin, taking you further than you expected underwater into a different and more challenging arena. This is not doilies and lavender bags: this is how to restructure your whole life. 'Make a friend of your worst enemy. Make the first advances, try desperately to understand their point of view . . . Do not be afraid to humble yourself . . . Stop thinking about yourself. Think of the other person all the time . . . The woman who believes in "speaking her mind" or "calling a spade a spade" is never charming . . . Never make anyone feel hurt, angry, indignant or embarrassed by anything you may say or do either deliberately or thoughtlessly . . . ' These are the tough tenets Miss Ascroft lays down, along with painting your toenails and practising how to smile. Although some of the examples she gives are so old-fashioned as to be ridiculous ('Keep your curls brushed and combed and tied up in a pretty ribbon to match your nightdress') they are also thought-provoking and touching. Searching for beauty, being scrupulously clean, avoiding gossip: these feel like ancient wisdoms, not much admired at the moment but certain to re-emerge as the pendulum swings.

Who was Eileen Ascroft? A Miss Marple-ish spinster deploring the behaviour of the young? Well, first she was the wife of a film director and then afterwards she became Mrs Hugh Cudlipp, at the heart of the Fleet Street elite; while he was Chairman of the Mirror Group she introduced a daily woman's page to the *Evening Standard*, no mean feat in those hard-boiled, male-dominated days of publishing. She was blonde, talented and reputedly snobbish and ambitious. Their lifestyle was cushioned by housekeepers, secretaries and chauffeurs; they seemed an enviable couple. But the Cudlipps had blazing rows and extra-marital affairs, and by the time Eileen was planning to leave him ('I feel I've done all I can for Hugh') he had already fallen for a colleague and friend of hers. Eileen's death by an accidental overdose of sleeping pills (she wrote in her last note to her husband: 'I had to try & get some sleep. As you know I haven't slept for nights . . .') seems a tragically long way from her advised method of achieving serenity: 'If at the end of the day you find yourself depressed, tired or nervy give yourself a lovely, deep, warm bath, and be really extravagant for once with your bath salts and scented talcum powder and wallow in the warm scented water. You'll sleep like a baby afterwards.'

These fourteen lessons on how to grasp the Magic Key to Charm are practical and inspiring. If they seem to yearn for impossibly high standards, maybe that's a challenge we can meet. Part of the path to charm may lie in gaily checked gingham overalls, a clear conscience and freely swinging arms. But look deeper: look inside yourself, arm yourself against 'all hurtful sordid things of the world . . . Hold your head up and be glad to be alive.' I will Miss Ascroft, and thank you very much.

Joanna Lumley, 2007

THE MAGIC KEY TO

- CHARM -

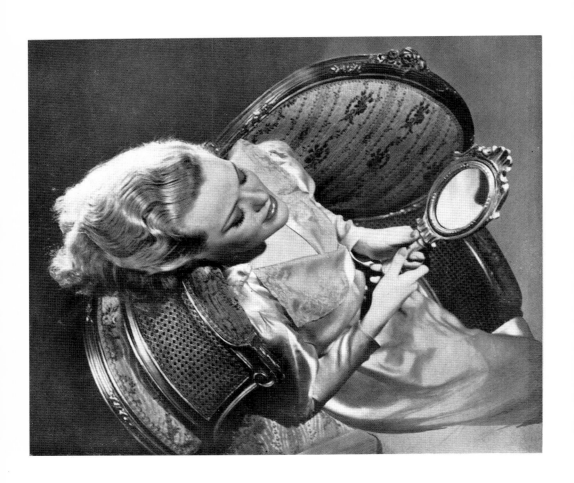

A NEW LIFE BEGINS

🙢   🙢   🙢

"A FLOWER without a perfume is like a personality without charm."

No woman, however beautiful or clever she may be, can live her life to the full unless she learns the secret of charm.

And every woman, no matter who she is, where she lives, what her age, or her job in life, can be charming.

Because charm lies already in her soul. She has only to learn how to set it free and express it to others.

Charm is every woman's birthright. It is a precious gift that God gives to each tiny baby girl when she first comes into the world.

Charm is there already in your soul. You have only to liberate it.

That is what we are going to do together in these lessons, learn how to express the charm that is already in you.

We are going to study together how to bring out the very best in you in three ways.

First, mentally, by directing your thoughts and actions into beautiful channels and filling your mind and brain so full of charming constructive thoughts that there will be no room for ugly, destructive ones.

Secondly, by practical advice about how to use clothes and make-up to emphasize your personality.

We are going to learn the importance of graceful movements and study how to walk and sit and run beautifully, and how to use our hands and care for our health and beauty.

And we are going to learn how to bring beauty into your home, too, and make it a truly charming setting for the charming person you are going to be.

And thirdly we are going to study your attitude to others together and learn how to find friendship and love.

YOU have become my pupil to-day.

Remember that word . . . to-day.

Make a note of its date in your personal diary, because to-day will begin to change your life.

To-day you are going to take stock of yourself.

To-day you are going to hold up a mirror before your own eyes and look into it frankly, honestly.

You are not only going to see your face in that mirror, your physical beauty ; you are going to see yourself as you really are. You—the eternal you.

For it is only then that we may realize the deeper lesson of these words of Keats :

"Beauty is truth, truth beauty—that is all
Ye know on earth, and all ye need to know."

YOU have probably longed at intervals in your life to make yourself a new woman—to be intelligent, poised, popular and beautiful.

Every woman who is worthy of the name of woman has pondered how she could bring into the world more radiance, more glamour.

How she could illuminate her home with joy and gaiety, how she could bring into the lives of her family and friends and of those around her some of the brilliance of the sun, the mellowness of the moon, some of the music of the trees, some of the captivating simplicity of the flowers.

You may have made little, half-hearted efforts about it and written out lists of good resolutions at the beginning of each new year.

And then, somehow, you forgot them all after a week or so, because you didn't seem to be getting anywhere.

That was because you were alone in your search. You didn't quite know what you wanted, you weren't sure how to go about getting it. You got discouraged and gave it up.

But now it is all going to be different.

You are no longer alone in your search.

I have promised to show you the way and work with you step by step until we reach your triumphant goal—*CHARM*.

To-NIGHT when you have shut your bedroom door against the outer world, when you are alone and at peace, face yourself in your mirror and say these words :

"I am going to be a new woman. Not beautiful, unless God gave me Beauty. Not glamorous unless I was born with Glamour. To-day I am going to be a new woman . . . a woman with *CHARM*."

And to-day it will begin to happen. To you. Do not be surprised and do not make a mistake ; I am not going to teach you tricks— I know none.

I am not going to show you how to produce something from your hat as a conjurer produces rabbits—and try to solve the mystery of charm in that way.

Because, you see, there is no mystery about charm.

Remember you have charm already. I am only going to show you how to show everyone else that you have that charm.

REMEMBER that. The soul is yours. What I am going to give you is the Magic Key to the soul.

And you are going to learn—patiently, step by step—how that Magic Key can open for you the doors that you have imagined until now were to be closed to you for ever.

There is the door of Friendship that I am going to open for you with this Magic Key.

And the door of Happiness too.

And greatest of all—the door of Love.

Every woman has known Love. The love of Mother for Babe. Of Babe for Mother. Of Girl for Boy. Of Woman for Man.

And every woman knows this, too ; that there is a love that is greater than all these things—the love of Life itself.

That love which brings to the very soul a warmth that it never knew before, that brings to your very inner heart a joy that before this wondrous moment it could only find in the illusion of a lovely dream.

EVERY now and then—sometimes among your friends—sometimes on the silver screen, sometimes on the stage—you see a woman who is "different," a woman who not only has Charm (as we all have) but who RADIATES charm.

And when you see her stroll nonchalantly into a drawing-room at a party, or into a scene on the stage—poised to perfection, dressed with so much delicacy that even the word "chic" itself seems a crude description of the subtlety and pleasing personality—you pause and wonder . . . "Could I ever be like that ? Could I ever be dressed so beautifully, could I ever smile with such content, and walk so gracefully, and talk so musically, and be in love—yes, in love—with Life itself ?"

I used to ask myself that question. Often—and searchingly.

And I learnt never to forget—that it is not only the flow of rich brocade or the warmth of crimson velvet, or the rustle of taffeta, or the joie de vivre of muslin and chiffon, that transforms a woman into a well-dressed queen.

Not only the wondrous mysteries of the beauty box that give a woman beauty ; not a perfect body that gives a woman poise. Not, not these things ; not one of them.

But simply—Charm.

To be charming you must be at peace with the world, and, still more important, with yourself.

For no woman who is at peace with herself will ever feel inferior or superior or self-conscious or affected in the presence of others.

Self-consciousness, affectedness, hate, pride and nervousness are all enemies of charm.

Are any of these faults spoiling your expression of charm ?

Ask yourself this question out loud : "Can I truthfully say that I am never self-conscious ?"

If the answer is yes, then ask yourself the same question again, substituting the word "affected" for "self-conscious." Then again substituting the word "hate," and so on.

But if the answer is no . . .

A self-conscious woman is a woman who does not know herself.

She has never faced herself quietly alone and discovered what sort of a person she really is.

She does not know what she wants from life or from other people —she does not know what she wants from herself.

If you admit you are self-conscious, that you are unsure of yourself and uncertain of how you appear in the eyes of other people—you must learn to know yourself.

Then you will no longer be uncertain.

Here is a valuable lesson that will show you how you can do this.

Close your eyes and make your mind a blank.

Then start to paint the picture of yourself in your mind substituting your own name and particulars.

Say, "I am Mary Ellen Smith——

"I am twenty-five years old——

"I have brown hair, blue eyes and a fair skin——

"I weigh 115 pounds and I am 5 ft. 4 in. tall——

"I work as a secretary in a big London office——

"I enjoy my work and am competent at my job——

"My hobbies are tennis and swimming in the summer and skating in winter——

"I like reading. I prefer light novels. Of all the books I read in the last year I liked *Gone with the Wind*, by Margaret Mitchell, best because I felt myself identified with the heroine, Scarlett O'Hara——

"My favourite colour is blue, the colour of the sky when the sun is at its most brilliant——

"My favourite flower is the sweet pea, because it makes me remember my mother's old-fashioned flower garden——

"My favourite piece of music is Beethoven's seventh Symphony because the wild soaring of the violins carries my soul away with ecstasy.

"My favourite song is 'Honey' because it brings back soft, shy memories of the first time I fell in love.

"My favourite poem is Wordsworth's 'She was a Phantom of Delight,' because it expresses in some elusive way the person I would like to be——"

Continue sketching in the picture of yourself, every detail you can think of.

Then, when you have the picture clearly in your mind, when it is finished, say to yourself : "This is me as I am and as the world sees me. I will not blurr this picture in future with self-doubt."

For when you are sure of yourself, there will be no room for self-doubt and self-consciousness will disappear.

IF you admit that you are affected, do the same exercise as for self-consciousness.

Know yourself and be true to that self and affectedness will have no part in your make-up.

And hate——

I have promised to give you the Magic Key that will open the door for you to Friendship, Happiness and LOVE.

But where there is hate, love cannot enter.

The best way to send hate out of your life is to make up your mind to make a friend of your worst enemy.

Make the first advances, try desperately to understand their point of view.

Do not be afraid to humble yourself. For in true humility there is strength.

Do not cease your efforts until you can call that person a friend—until all those whom you now feel antagonistic to or who feel antagonistic to you are your friends.

And to get rid of pride. Follow the same exercise as for self-consciousness.

For pride is just another form of self-doubt.

Nervousness is perhaps the greatest enemy of all to Charm. Nervous habits, nervous mannerisms of speech, loss of control.

The charming woman must have perfect control at all times.

Ask yourself honestly : "Have I any nervous habits which may be irritating to others and which reveal that I have not full self-control ?"

These questions will help you to find out.

1. Do I bite my nails or pick at them when they lie in my lap?
2. Do I frequently pat my hair or twist curls into place?
3. Do I fidget with jewellery?
4. Do I swing my foot or tap it on the floor when sitting?
5. Do I rub my hands as if I were washing them?
6. Do I pick at things with my fingers?
7. Do I fidget with my clothes?
8. Do I touch my face frequently?
9. Do I scratch my head?
10. Do I snap my suspenders or pull down my suspender belt?
11. Do I clear my throat nervously before speaking?
12. Do I stutter?
13. Do I repeat myself?
14. Have I got a nervous, affected giggle?
15. At table, do I fiddle with the cutlery or glasses?
16. Do I crumble my bread or roll it into little balls?
17. When reading, do I twist the corners of the pages nervously?
18. Have I a nervous cough?
19. Do I pull at my ear lobes?
20. Do I hum nervously under my breath?

*C*AN *you honestly say that you have none of these nervous habits ?*
If you can, so much the better.
If you can't, you must get rid of them.
For each one is an enemy of charm.
You know how ugly they are in other people and how irritating they appear. They appear just the same in you to others.

Watch yourself in front of your mirror and you'll see how ugly they are.

Self-control, of course, can banish any of them and you must exert it to the full, but there are several other little things that will assist you.

Ask your family to help you by telling you when you do it.

You probably don't always realize when you are doing it yourself and they'll be quick enough to tell you.

Ask your best friends to help. Make it a joke and they'll laugh you out of it !

To stop biting your nails, have them manicured in a shop for a while and shame yourself into growing them.

Try wearing bright red polish, then every time you lift your fingers to your mouth, you'll see red !

Try covering your hands with nourishing cream and sleeping in cotton gloves.

It'll stop you biting your nails and make your hands soft and white as well.

Nervousness of speech can be cured by always thinking before you speak and speaking more slowly.

Your hands seem to be the chief offenders.

When you are not using your hands, always keep them relaxed in your lap or on the arm of the chair.

When next you catch them fidgeting, do this little exercise to relax them :—

Hold them up, palms facing, a little away from each other. Now stretch them as hard as you can, from the elbows, right down to the finger-tips.

Now relax them completely and let your fingers curl softly down on to your palms.

Do this three times, then let them lie softly in your lap.

The best cure for nervous coughs and giggles is to think of someone else you know who does it and to exert every scrap of will-power not to make such a spectacle of yourself.

17

B

Don't be content until you can answer "No" with assurance to those twenty questions.   Remember each fault overcome is a stepping-stone across the river of ugliness to charm.

⚘

BESIDES learning to be at peace with yourself, with the world— you must honestly *approve* of yourself.

By this I mean there must be nothing about your behaviour or appearance which gives you the slightest feeling of shame.

Ask yourself these three questions every night before retiring :—

"Have I done to-day anything of which I feel ashamed?"

"Have I been kind and considerate to every person with whom I have been in contact to-day?"

"Have I done at least one thing to-day of which I can be a little proud?"

You may think this all sounds very smug and serious, but you must believe it is really necessary to have a clear conscience and an untroubled mind before you can develop the charm that lies within you.

For your soul is like a garden.

If the ground is sweet and clear and you plant lovely flowers of thought in it, they will grow and flourish.

But if you neglect the soil and allow little weeds of doubt and guilt to grow up, they will choke the flowers you try to plant.

So keep your conscience clear, your mind untroubled and seek as many beautiful things to think about as possible and lock their memories away in your heart.

⚘

BUY a book of beautiful poetry and read a poem each day, savouring the beauty and rhythm of the lines.

For it is from the simple appeal of beautiful words that you may discover some of the secret of charm itself.

LESSON TWO

SERENITY

    ✤   ✤   ✤

ALREADY, if you have carried out my advice, you have passed the first milestone on the road to charm.

That milestone is the simple realization of the fact that charm is something within your own soul.

Something that does not radiate from without to within, but something that glows from within to without.

The knowledge that Charm is no mystery, that it is something within the grasp of every woman.

Now in this lesson we are going to develop the charm that is in you, spiritually from within and practically from without.

✤

FIRST, I want you to stand or sit before your mirror and ask yourself these questions.

"Do I want to feel at ease in any company in which I may find myself?"

"Do I want people to like me instinctively when they meet me?"

"Do I want to be a cultured, interesting person?"

"Do I want to bring more charm into my voice—its pitch, accent and words?"

"Do I really want to know my body—its perfections and its flaws—so that I may develop every scrap of charm it possesses?"

19

"Do I want to think beautiful thoughts and be able to rid my mind of nagging, little worries ?"

"Do I want my smile to be a lovely, captivating thing ?"

"Do I want to know how to emphasize my personality with colour and clothes ?"

"Do I want all my movements to be naturally graceful ones ?"

"Do I want to be a charming wife—mother—daughter—sister ?"

"Do I want my home to be a perfect setting for my personality ?"

"Do I want to bring friendship and love into my life ?"

And to each of these questions you will answer YES.

For they embody all a woman wants from life.

You want all this and you can have it. When we come together to the end of this book, I shall have put the means into your hands. You have only to take it.

⁕

THE first step is to achieve daintiness and charm all around you, for you cannot be dainty and charming mentally if your physical surroundings are untidy and lacking in freshness and care.

Your clothes, your body, your own room, your personal possessions all must be spotlessly clean.

Cleanliness is the symbol of a fresh start.

Think how refreshing a hot bath at the end of a worrying day can be. Your troubles seem to melt away and you feel strong and fresh afterwards, ready to face the world once more.

That is how it must be with everything you possess.

Fastidiousness about your physical surroundings will help you to think in the same way.

Look round your room now and take stock of it carefully.

Is it spotlessly clean ? Is its colour scheme a charming background for you ? Do its brasses shine, are its curtains fresh and crisp, is its bedcover smooth, is everything tidy, is the linen snowy white ?

Now look again.

Is there anything in it that jars on you mentally, such as a china ornament or a picture, which you have always loathed, but somehow never discarded ?

If there is, take it away ruthlessly.

And now I want you to put something lovely into your room, something that gives you pleasure to look at it.

A reproduction of a beautiful picture perhaps, that will make you catch your breath with the wonderment of a little child.

A single rose in a slim, crystal vase, on your dressing table, which will give you a sense of luxury and beauty as you sit at your toilet.

Always try to sit at your dressing table when you are making up your face or brushing your hair. It gives one a luxurious, unhurried feeling.

Your room should be an intimate friend—a place where you can relax completely, pleasing to the eye, with beauty to refresh the soul.

Now go through your wardrobe, every single thing you wear and use, and make sure it is spotlessly clean, freshly pressed and repaired.

Remember an old dress, which has been carefully and lovingly tended, can be just as charming as any new frock.

And what about the drawers and cupboards in which you keep your clothes ? Are they lined with clean paper ? Are they freshly aired and not stuffy, smelling of cigarette smoke ?

Are your shoes on trees and your dresses and coats on individual hangers ? Are your handbags wrapped carefully in tissue paper ? Has everything its special place ?

Cover your coat-hangers with material of your favourite colour and hang a tiny lavender bag on each.

Tuck lavender bags among your clothes and keep one under your pillow to lend fragrance to your dreams.

Banish all that is ugly from you.   Surround yourself with things you love and which please your eyes.

I do not mean that you should scrap everything you have and buy new.   That would be expensive and foolish.

A vase of flowers, a delicately-scented talcum powder, your powder in a lovely coloured bowl instead of its box, your perfume in a coloured scent spray to match—all these little things bring charm into your surroundings and your life.

They make you pleased, happy, careful of the charm that is within you.

A VERY important thing—one of the first things we must learn together—is serenity.

The feeling of being at peace with yourself and with the whole world.   SERENITY.

Most people get nervy, worked up, irritable, anxious sometimes. It is the outcome of the hectic, unnatural life they live.

They rush about in trains and buses and crowds, with noise all around them.   Their nerves get jangled and taut.

And then little lines of strain creep into their face, their voice betrays their nervousness and Charm flies a million miles away.

The charming woman has an inner serenity, which is unaffected by circumstances.   She is always poised and gracious.

You never find her ruffled or bad tempered.

She has discovered the secret of serenity.

And you must discover the secret, too, and make it your own if you would discover the still more precious secret of Charm.

Now, in future, whenever you feel your nerves straining, when you feel irritable or a little, nagging worry keeps recurring in your mind, I want you to do this if the circumstances make it possible.

Sit still, lean back and relax. Relax utterly and completely. Let your limbs go limp.

Sink down into the chair and shut your eyes. Make your mind a blank and then think of a piece of rich, black velvet.

Concentrate on this until you are actually gazing into its deep, rich texture and hold this image in your mind's eye as long as you can.

You may think this sounds silly. I did when it was first told to me by a world-famous beauty specialist.

But I tried it and was amazed at the way it helped me to relax.

After that, whenever I began to feel nervy, worried or "tied up in knots" mentally, I used to do this little exercise. It only takes a few minutes.

If you find yourself in circumstances which make it impossible to do this exercise, draw in a deep breath and let it out slowly, at the same time making your mind blank for a few seconds.

And now make this resolution to-day :

"I am not going to worry. Worry does much harm and no good. In future I will not worry."

THERE is a very old saying : "When you meet trouble, count your blessings."

I am a firm believer in this. When the world's black and the out-look for to-morrow is depressing, one is apt to become self-pitying.

And what better antidote could there be to self-pity than to count one's blessings ?

Keep your eyes and ears open to beauty. Look for beauty in everything.

If you live near a picture gallery go there sometimes and study the beautiful paintings.   Try to absorb some of their beauty and colouring and line into your own mind.

Go for walks in the country. Look at the flowers, the trees, the earth and the insects.

Listen to the lovely song of the birds ; let your eyes feast on the rich wealth of colour.

Walk by the river if you live in London, and watch the swans gliding gracefully over the smooth surface of the water, arching their beautiful necks and beating their powerful wings.

If you pass a flower shop on your way to work, linger at the window and drink in the exquisite colour and form of the blooms.

Look at the marvellous colouring and texture of materials when you are shopping.

How often do you throw your head back and look up at the sky ? At the variations in blues and greys and purples, at the clouds, small and white and fleecy, or billowing and smudged with grey.

Fill your mind with lovely thoughts and beautiful memories. Then when the world is dark and cheerless, you can think of these things and be happy in their beauty.

SERENITY—Charm. The two words have the same beauty of sound.

If you have serenity, you have charm—if you have charm, you have serenity.

You cannot be serene if you are always hurried and flustered.

Try to banish hurry from your life. Give yourself a chance to live your life to the full.

It may be a busy life, and if it is, it will need planning all the more carefully so that you never feel worried or worn-out.

Never keep up full steam all day. Take a little time off for relaxation—complete relaxation.

If you have had a busy day and you are going out in the evening, lie down on your bed for at least ten minutes in a dark room.

Take off all your clothes and relax completely. Put two tiny pads

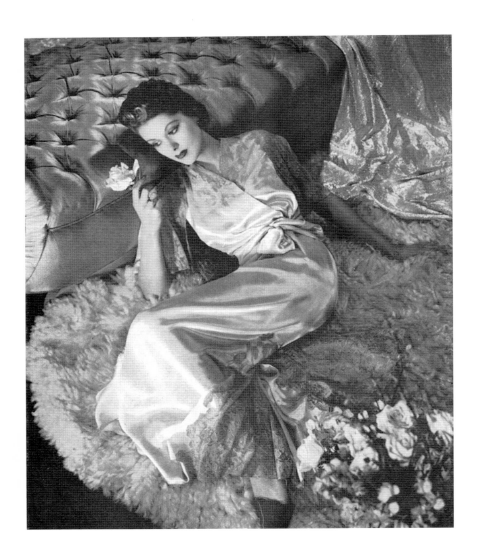

of cotton-wool, soaked in astringent, over your eyes. Then make your mind blank.

When you get up to dress after this you'll be feeling a new person.

If at the end of the day you find yourself depressed, tired or nervy, give yourself a lovely, deep, warm bath, and be really extravagant for once with your bath salts and scented talcum powder and wallow in the warm, scented water.

You'll sleep like a baby afterwards.

Always try to spend at least a quarter of an hour during the day relaxing and resting, if possible with your feet up and your eyes closed.

If you can't do that, just sit still for the same time, relaxing as much as possible especially in your thoughts.

So far we have spoken only of your attitude to yourself. But now we must talk of your attitude to other people.

Because half the little, nagging thoughts that harass your mind arise out of your reactions to others.

If you find yourself in contact with someone who is jealous of you or antagonistic towards you, do not be resentful towards them. And do not be offended or hurt either.

I know this may seem difficult sometimes, but it is very important because of its effect on you.

Remember that the other person has as much *inherent charm* as you have. The only difference is that you are learning to liberate Charm, to express it and to call it forth in others, too.

So meet antagonism with kindness—not condescension, but real simple kindness.

They are jealous because they feel you have something that they have not.

25

So make them pleased with something about themselves and their jealousy will disappear. Choose the most admirable thing about them and praise them for it.

If your praise is genuine they will respond to you and unkind thoughts will vanish.

You cannot afford to have enemies. Nobody can. They may never harm you directly, but the unspoken enmity between you will do harm enough by its inward effect.

Never try to impose your will on another person. Never nag, bully, threaten or despise someone because she doesn't agree with you.

Remember it is just as much your business to understand *her*.

There is a lovely charm about a woman who doesn't take offence, who doesn't gossip maliciously, who is naturally sweet-tempered.

YOU may say, "That's all very well, but I'm naturally quick-tempered. I can't help it."

But you can and must.

If you fill your mind with lovely thoughts and memories, there will be no room for vicious, destructive ones.

Be constructive. Give your mind things to think about. An idle mind gets into mischief just as an idle child does.

Never do anything of which you are ashamed or which you have to conceal, for when there is anything, large or small, on your conscience it will leave its mark on your face.

The tiny, sensitive muscles round your mouth will betray your thoughts and spoil the serenity of your expression.

Each temptation resisted, each tiny triumph of character, will leave its good influence on your face.

DISCOVER YOUR TYPE

CHARM—"If you have it, you don't need to have anything else. If you haven't, it doesn't matter what else you have." This is what the famous author, J. M. Barrie, said of charm.

It is a lovely saying. But there is one thing about which he is wrong. There is no woman without charm.

It is the birthright of every woman to be charming, poised, attractive, no matter what her age, her race, or her social position.

Every woman you meet whom you dismiss as dowdy, dull and colourless has charm buried in her soul.

Sometimes she doesn't know it's there and sometimes she doesn't know how to express it.

She does not know herself as she really is, she does not know the art of self-expression or the meaning of the word "personality."

Do not smother the charm that is within you. Unfold it. Do not make a mockery of your hidden beauty. Unfold it.

Learn to analyse the lovely, exciting person that is the inner you.

Only by knowing yourself thoroughly and being true to that self can you develop personality.

FROM my experience, I have discovered that there are seven theme types into which all women fall.

By the word "type" I do not mean that all women of one type have all the same characteristics.

That would be absurd.

No two women in the world are exactly alike.

Each has her own variations just as a Beethoven symphony has many variations on the same theme.

It is the theme that is the same. So let us call them, then, the seven "theme types."

It is necessary that you understand what type you belong to if you are to unfold within yourself the greatest possible degree of charm from the lessons on beauty, dress and the home which I will be giving you soon.

Which theme type are you? Read through them all and discover which is yours. You will find the physical characteristics of each type a helpful guide, as each type is decided by her glandular arrangement.

THE MATERNAL TYPE is a very usual type that rules the world by rocking more cradles than any other type.

You have a figure better suited to Edwardian times than the very slim silhouettes of the present day.

Your face is the Madonna type, oval in shape, with a clear, smooth skin and a good colour.

You are swayed entirely by your emotions, which are primarily maternal and you think with your heart.

You fall in love **very** deeply, but whether you know it or not, you are sub-consciously searching for a good father for your children.

You are a very conventional type and you can always be relied upon to do the right thing.

You make a very good wife who is always faithful to her husband.

You are wonderfully loyal to your friends and family and would give the last drop of your heart's blood for your children.

In fact, you are over-anxious for their welfare. You are inclined to smother them with attention, to try to think and act for them.

You are inclined to take offence rather easily and become embroiled in petty quarrels and arguments. This is something you must curb in yourself.

It reveals a lack of poise, of self-confidence. It is most important for you to cultivate serenity.

For you are fundamentally the Madonna type, the symbol of peaceful beauty and tender motherhood.

You have the secret charm in you to make your home into a little haven of peace and happiness for your family.

THE MAN'S GIRL is cheery, a good sort, very kind to the underdog and foolishly generous.

Your figure is usually well-developed.

Your skin is fine, clear, moist and pink-and-white.

Your mouth is wide and the lips voluptuously curved.

Your hair almost always has blonde tendencies.

You are usually in great demand with the menfolk, but more for an evening's fun than as a wife and mother.

Though you are good-tempered as a general rule, you are given to flaring up into sudden tempers when you give way to your feelings and say many things you regret afterwards.

Beware of these tempers. Your chief charm is your kind, generous good humour.

You enjoy a little flirtation, but you soon grow tired and look round for variety.

If you marry, you will be very kind to your husband and children. They will love you for your gaiety and good humour.

You are inclined to be rather philosophical in a live-and-let-live manner.

It is charming when it portrays itself in an affection for all the world and everyone in it and a willingness to extend a helping hand to anyone in need of it.

But beware of being lazy about yourself.

You have the possibilities of a wonderful friend, loyal, cheerful, generous, kind-hearted.

THE CLEVER TYPE is logical, clear-thinking and level-headed.

You are usually either very tall or very short.

Your hair is fair and fine, rather apt to be colourless, probably a dead, ashy tone.

You have a mature, individual outlook on life and you are quick to assimilate new ideas.

You have a wonderful memory and have the unusual gift in a woman of being able to profit by experience.

You are excellent in business, reliable and efficient and invariably make a success of your job.

You are intensely independent, you think for yourself and allow no one to influence you unduly.

In fact, you are a little too headstrong, rather inclined to ride rough-shod over others, often hurting their feelings in the process.

You have great courage, due to a combination of self-control and clear-sightedness.

You often take great risks, but you always know what you are letting yourself in for.

Your head rules your heart completely. You always consider the pro's and con's before falling in love.

In fact, you are inclined to be too hard and calculating and need to cultivate the softer, sweeter side of your nature.

Love is not a very important factor in your life.

You will be a loyal, intelligent wife, but the mother instinct is not very strong.

You are fundamentally the gallant, clever type. You can carry responsibility, and have infinite self-control and great loyalty. And in your eyes shines the true light of courage.

※

THE PERFECT WIFE is a very feminine person. You are every mother's dream wife for her son.

You are usually well-proportioned, slender.

You have delicate features, a gentle, serene expression, a smooth, moist skin, beautiful silky hair, often straight, frequently dark.

You are gentle, graceful, poised and reserved. You are well-balanced, mentally and physically, and you have a great fund of nervous energy, which you know how to use and how to control.

You are usually pleasing in appearance, softly pretty, with dreams in your eyes.

You often have artistic leanings, but you make a success of almost any work you undertake, especially if it is creative.

You are very unselfish and sympathetic. You can be relied upon to stand by anyone in a tight spot.

You like men's company and you get on very well with them but you subconsciously dread the moment when that certain light comes into their eyes.

Nevertheless, when you do marry you usually make an excellent wife and mother, for you will never cease your efforts to make your marriage successful.

※

THE GOOD TIME GIRL has heaps of nervous energy and is rather lacking in self-control.

Perhaps your most characteristic feature is your eyes, which are extremely prominent, large, brilliant, burning with a "what next?" expression, and have unusually long eyelashes.

Your skin is smooth, delicate and pale, with perhaps a slight flush over the cheekbones.

Your hair is full of life and vitality, thick, usually brunette, sometimes of an exquisite and unusual dark red.

Your whole character is restless. You want constant variety all the time, but you are never quite sure what you want to do next.

You have considerable artistic ability, and if you could only stabilize yourself a bit you would make a success of a creative job.

But you are a lovely butterfly and rarely stick at anything long.

You are a slave to your moods, always exquisitely elated or depressed.

For this reason you do not make a very good wife, unless you practise great control and your husband is a very balanced person.

It would really be better for you not to have children as you are not the mother type and would not provide a stable home background for them.

You are too irresponsible to be held by any chains, even domestic ones.

Men will adore you for your vitality, and the vivacious beauty which is nearly always yours. Many of them will fall passionately in love with you.

But you will never be really happy unless you cultivate an inner serenity, unless you are capable of being at peace with yourself and the world sometimes.

THE CHILDISHLY APPEALING TYPE has rather childish features and all the charm of a child.

You may be any height, but you will be slim and rounded and appear almost boneless.

Your complexion is your best feature ; it is translucent, and delicately coloured.

Your eyes are big and innocent, often blue, and you have a tiny nose, which may be retroussée.

You are a feminine Peter Pan. But in spite of your eternally youthful spirit you have a mind of your own and amazing strength of purpose.

You know very clearly what you want from life and how to get it and you have little conscience.

You are inclined to be selfish and a little unscrupulous about things you want.

You're not much interested in men, except as a means for a good time.

You are very sweet to your women friends as long as they do not try to oppose you.

You are fun to be with and you have plenty of high spirits.

You make a good wife for a rather paternal type of man, usually several years your senior.

He will love your youthful spirits and probably spoil you shamelessly and you will love it !

Don't let materialism spoil the charm of your youthful appeal or a calculating look replace the wistful wonder in your eyes.

THE GLAMOROUS TYPE is vivacious and has a lot of sheer animal spirits.

Your eyes are quick and darting—probably brown. Your mouth is large with rather thick lips.

Your hair is coarse, dry, full of electricity ; often curly ; often of unusual colour—jet black, corn gold, bright red.

You are usually strong, with great stamina and very energetic. You are rather hot-tempered and sometimes aggressive, which causes you unhappiness.

C

You are ruthless and tireless and often do well in business where you have scope for your considerable organizing abilities.

Your imagination is usually strong and you have a nice little sense of intrigue.

You have great control of your body. You are good at games and probably dance, ride and swim well.

You are usually fairly interested in sex and although you are not a lot impressed by "being in love," you often have many romances both before and after marriage.

You like to be popular and the centre of attraction. You make a good wife as long as you live up to the highest that is in you, and your husband usually goes far through your help and push.

You are a good mother and bring your children up to be useful, healthy citizens.

You want to curb that too ready temper that flares up to spoil the charm of your character.

Try to be a little more considerate of others and realize this—that sex and love must be one and the same thing in their highest, most lovely forms.

Love without sex is like a plant with no flowers. Sex without love is like an artificial flower.

BEAUTY

❧   ❧   ❧

IN our last lessons together, we made a thrilling discovery.

We found the real you. We discovered the kind of person you were meant to be and, more important, the kind of person you could become.

We made a clear sketch together of what we want to achieve with you, the things we want to develop, others which we need to change or eradicate altogether.

But the sketch of the charming person you are going to be is clearly there. Keep it in mind all through this course.

Now we are going to colour that picture, in beautiful shades. We are going to give it many tones of light and shade. And the picture is going to be a masterpiece.

In this chapter we are going to speak of cosmetics and beauty treatments, and how to use them to bring out every scrap of natural beauty in your face.

Cosmetics should never be used to hide, only to enhance what is already there.

No cosmetics on earth will hide the unpleasant signs in a face of a spiteful, bitter soul.

No lipstick can disguise a cruel twist to a mouth, no eye shadow or mascara hides calculating eyes and no creams or foundations the lines of discontent and bitterness in a face.

The only way to banish these blemishes is from within.

35

Substitute kind thoughts for bitter ones, generosity for meanness, understanding for hardness, for everything that goes on within reveals itself in your face.

SOME women think it is a waste of time or pandering to vanity to spend too much time on their faces.

How wrong they are!

The world needs beauty and charm. There is enough ugliness all around us to-day.

It is up to each woman to make herself as physically beautiful as she is able.

It is her duty to the world and to herself.

She avails herself of every modern invention to make her house more beautiful and more efficient.

So why should she be ashamed of using every modern invention to enhance the loveliness of her face?

Every face needs a good foundation, powder, lipstick; some faces need rouge, eyebrow pencil and mascara also.

Every face needs a good morning and evening routine and usually a face mask once a week. Here are simple home treatments I have worked out for the dry, normal and greasy skins :—

Morning routine for the normal skin.

Cleanse thoroughly with a good cleansing cream and remove with face tissues. Follow this with a mild astringent. If you use water on your face, be sure to use a good bland soap and to rinse well in cold water afterwards.

Smooth on a little foundation cream, then apply either a powder or a cream rouge and powder over it.

Night routine for the normal skin.

Cleanse thoroughly with a good cleansing cream and remove with face tissues. If you use water on your face, use a good bland soap.

If you are young, use a nourishing skin food about twice a week, massage it into the skin, then blot off the surplus with tissues.

If you are over thirty-five, use a skin food every night, especially round the eyes.

Face mask for the normal skin.

Take a dessertspoonful of fuller's-earth and mix with white of an egg, a few drops of lemon juice and enough milk to make a creamy paste.

Cleanse your face thoroughly, then spread on the pack and leave for about a quarter of an hour.

Lie down if possible and relax while the mask is on. Rinse it off with warm water afterwards.

Morning routine for the greasy skin.

Thoroughly cleanse with complexion milk, then apply a good astringent with a pad of cotton-wool. If you use water on your face, be sure to use a good bland soap and rinse in cold water afterwards.

Now smooth a powder lotion evenly over your face and neck.

If you use rouge, you will find a powder rouge better than a greasy one. Apply before powdering.

Night routine for the greasy skin.

Cleanse the face thoroughly with complexion milk. If you use water on your face, use a good bland soap and rinse well in cold water afterwards.

It is better not to use cream on the face if your skin is very greasy.

Face mask for the greasy skin.

If your skin is coarse and oily, use this face pack at least once a week.

Beat up plain white of egg in a basin and then spread it over the face. It dries very quickly.

Let it dry thoroughly and stay on for about a quarter of an hour before removing it with cold water.

Morning routine for the dry skin.

Thoroughly cleanse with a good cleansing cream and remove with face tissues. Follow with a very mild astringent. If you use water on your face, use a good almond oil soap and rinse well with cold water afterwards.

Apply a really nourishing powder base. Then, if you use rouge, a cream one is best for you.

Apply a very little to each cheek and blend it into the skin gently. Then powder over it.

Night routine for the dry skin.

Cleanse the face thoroughly with a good cleansing cream. If you use water on your face choose a good almond oil soap.

Now pat on more cleansing cream and leave on while you bath. Then remove the cream with face tissues and massage a rich, nourishing cream into the skin and leave on all night.

Face mask for the dry skin.

Make a butter muslin mask of two thicknesses, with strings to tie round your head and neck and holes for eyes and nose.

Then mix equal quantities of almond and mineral oils together and heat.

Now mix six drops of tincture of benzoin with four drams of your favourite toilet water and mix this with the oil.

Cleanse your face well first with cleansing cream and then smear the oil all over the face and neck with your finger-tips.

Now dip the mask in the oil and cover the face with it.

Lie down and rest now, and leave the mask on as long as possible.

When you take it off, wipe the surplus oil off with face tissues, then with cotton-wool pads dipped in astringent.

THESE masks can all be made very cheaply at home, but there are many excellent ones on the market already prepared for use.

If you can afford a little money now and then to spend on your face visit a beauty salon and have a professional face treatment.

Besides keeping the skin of your face in good condition you must use the right shades of cosmetics to suit your colouring, and bring out the greatest beauty in your face. And you must learn how to use them to get the best results. Here are some general make-up rules which will help you.

1. Never alter the shape of your eyebrows without consulting an expert.

   Nature designed the shape of your brows to suit the rest of your face. If you alter them you may spoil the character of your face.

   It is better just to tidy up the stray hairs with eyebrow pluckers, or thin them a little if they are too thick.

2. Don't use rouge as a matter of course. Nature may have intended you to be fragilely pale.

3. If you use rouge, make sure you apply it rightly. It should never show in a hard line on the cheeks, but be softly blended right into the skin so that it gives a natural bloom.

   If you have a long, thin face, apply your rouge fairly high up under the eyes and blend it outwards towards the outer edges of the face. This will give your face width.

   But if your face is round in contour, you can narrow it by applying your rouge close in to the nose.

4. When making up your mouth, blot off the surplus lipstick with a face tissue. Place it between the lips and close them

over it. A lip pencil is helpful for outlining the shape of the mouth.

5. Always apply mascara under the lashes, brushing them upwards.

   A much more natural effect is achieved by darkening just the upper lashes. This also makes the eyes appear larger.

   There is a good little gadget called Kurlash for curling up straight lashes. In two seconds it gives them that lovely starry look.

6. If you use an eyebrow pencil, use it just on the hairs of the brows. Be careful not to draw on the skin, as this gives a hard line.

7. When you powder, put it on fairly thickly with a fresh pad of cotton-wool each time.

   Leave it for a minute, then dust off the surplus with a little powder brush.

   You will find it will stay on much longer and give a lovely matt effect this way.

   Always use a clean powder puff as soon as one gets the slightest bit soiled.

8. If your face is long and narrow, a lighter powder on the cheeks often helps to widen it.

   In the same way, a round, fat face, with a small nose, can be lengthened with a lighter powder on the nose, chin and forehead, and a big nose can be subdued with a darker powder than the rest of the face.

NOW here is an exercise I want you to perform to-night before you go to bed.

Shut yourself alone in your bedroom and study your face.

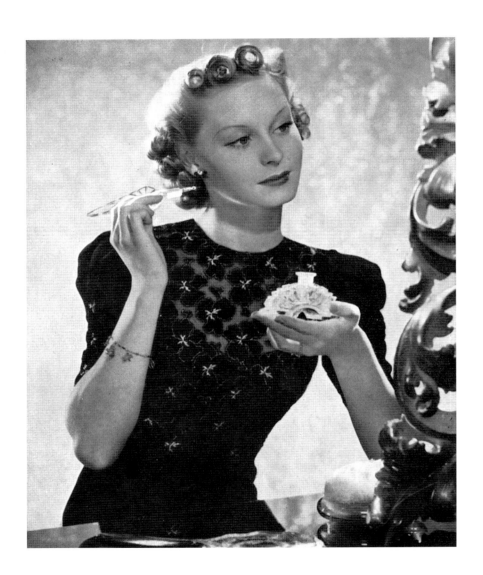

For your face is the key to what you really are. It is written there for all the world to see.

Look at all the tiny lines on it (I'm not referring to wrinkles !)—at the little lines from nose to mouth caused by laughter.

Though you will try to smooth these out with nourishing creams and massage, for the sake of the outward beauty of your face, there is no real need to worry about these lines. They do not spoil the charm of your face.

They tell the world that you are a happy person, a kind person, someone who is always ready to look on the bright side of things.

Now look at your forehead—at the tiny lines of discontent and worry.

Those are the lines you want to banish—must banish.

Say to yourself, "I am going to stop worrying and being discontented. It gets me nowhere and it sketches little tell-tale lines on my face.

"I will keep a book of lovely poems or a beautiful book to read when I start to worry or feel discontented.

"I will remember the loveliest thing I have ever seen, a sunset over water, a rainbow in the country, a snow scene at Christmas, but I will stop worrying and feeling discontented."

One thing that I think is important is to keep all your aids to beauty beautiful.

Keep one drawer in your dressing-table as your make-up drawer.

I have lined mine with rose-pink American cloth, fixed in with pink drawing-pins.

Then I can wipe it over every so often and keep it fresh and clean.

I keep everything in separate little boxes, my manicure things all together, my face tissues and my cotton-wool all in their own containers.

I think a good rule to keep about all your personal possessions is this : Keep everything about you so fresh and so dainty that if your most fastidious acquaintance were to ask to borrow anything you could lend it to her without any apologies or embarrassment.

41

And now we come to your body. What do you really know about this body of yours, of its shape, its texture, its power?

Have you ever studied it? Have you ever looked at yourself unclothed in a long mirror?

Do it to-night, when you are all alone and at peace with the world, when the troubles of the day have faded in the twilight.

Do it again to-morrow night, and again the next night until any embarrassment you may feel at first no longer exists.

For it is very silly to be ashamed of your body.

Many women are, and they must learn to lose this shame.

For how can you be true to yourself if you are afraid to face that self, afraid to know that self?

Look at the beauty of that body God has given you.

At your hair, your face, your eyes, which reflect your soul.

Look at the rhythmic curve of your shoulders, the exquisite soft whiteness of your breasts.

Look at the beauty of your thighs, at the classic curves of your legs as they taper and taper just as the stems of a flower.

There can be no self-deception between you and yourself when you are standing in the nude.

You see yourself as God made you. You can't help but be awed by the beauty of His work.

IT is not enough to know and appreciate the beauty of your body. You must also learn to preserve its flowerlike beauty.

Keep it always spotlessly clean and fresh.

Always see that all your toilet things have the same perfume, as conflicting scents can often kill each other's beauty.

Unless your skin is greasy, it will need an occasional nourishment to keep its lovely soft texture.

So about once a week, after a hot bath, rub a little almond oil all over it and massage it well in.

Give your toes a weekly pedicure when you do your manicure, and if you use a coloured nail varnish, paint your toes to match your finger-tips.

It's very good for one's self-esteem to see ten pink shining beautifully groomed toes peeping up from the bath water.

Your hands are very important and deserve attention, for this reason : they reveal your character just as clearly as your eyes.

From people's hands you can always tell what sort of people they are.

So keep yours soft and white with a good hand cream, used every time after you wash.

If you use a nail varnish, always see that it is immaculate.

If you don't, keep your finger-tips beautifully polished with a nail buffer.

And remember your hands express you, so encourage them to express the best that is in you.

Practise lovely gestures, moving them gracefully and unhurriedly.

Watch the hands of actresses or film stars, and you will see that hands can be beautiful to watch even when engaged in homely little tasks like knitting or emptying a saucepan.

KEEP your hair bright and shining as it was intended to be. If it is dull or lifeless, find out the cause and cure it.

Ask your hairdresser, and if he can't help you, consult your doctor.

A weekly shampoo will keep it soft and pretty and, if it is inclined to be dry, give it an occasional warm oil bath the night before you shampoo it.

When choosing the perfect hairdressing for you, there are three things to consider :—

1. Your personality, your type.

2. What sort of life you lead.
3. Shapes of features.

Never adopt a hair-style unless you are sure it is right for you and you feel happy and at ease with it, and remember it's much more important to keep the hair beautifully groomed than to wear the latest style.

I CONSIDER it is a woman's duty to keep the body God gave her lovely to look at.

And I also think it her duty to keep that same body in proper working order, for there is no greater enemy to beauty and charm than ill-health.

One important thing to remember is that Good Health is Natural.

Only by abusing our bodies or contracting some disease do we have bad health.

I have spoken with many doctors about the essential rules to keep a woman in good health, and I give here ten simple rules for health :—

1. Never take medicines unless you have to.
2. Try to get the same amount of sleep each night, be it six hours, seven, eight or nine.
3. Stick to a well-balanced diet, no food fads.
4. Don't over-eat. Don't under-eat.
5. See your dentist every six months.
6. Drink about two pints of liquid a day.
7. Spotless cleanliness.
8. Avoid infection as far as possible.
9. Sleep with your windows open.
10. Take a moderate amount of exercise.

CLOTHES

🙢   🙢   🙢

Now that you have learned what Charm is, you must learn how to express it.

In your voice, in your movements, in your actions, in your possessions and in your appearance.

We are going to talk about your appearance in this lesson, the outward you that must express the inner you.

Remember that many people never have the chance of meeting the inner you and they will judge you on the way you look.

That is why clothes and the way you wear them are so important.

They are one of your chief means of putting your personality across to the world.

So many women make the mistake of trying to suit their personality to their clothes.

One night they will wear a demure Victorian gown with ringlets and the next night a slim, sheath-like dress with a daring décolletage and a sophisticated hair-style.

Both dresses may be lovely in themselves. But one of those frocks, or maybe both, is not expressing her personality.

She is sinking her own individuality in that of her clothes and she is forfeiting Charm because of it.

Here and now I want you to make a solemn vow to yourself. I want you to say these words out loud.

"In future I am going to dress only to express myself. I am never going to buy anything just because it is fashionable or because it is a bargain.

"Everything I wear is going to express my personality and my personal Charm to the world."

IN the third lesson, you remember how we discovered your personality together, by analysing your theme type?

We decided you were one of seven basic theme types. Though, of course, you have many variations of your own, just as in a piece of music there are many variations on the same theme.

And now you want to know how best to express that personality —your personality—in your clothes.

The following advice for each theme type will help you.

MATERNAL TYPE.—Yours are all the lovely soft stuffs and pastel shades to express your sweet, feminine self.

If you like flowers wear them. Choose the ones you love and which hold something for you.

Roses, violets, stephanotis are a perfect expression of your fragrant charm.

In the daytime wear them in a little knot tucked into your waistband or in your hat.

In the evening get your florist to make you a flower bracelet with a piece of ribbon to match your frock.

Don't wear a low décolletage, or anything too eccentric. They are the exact opposite of that inner charm we—yes, you and I, are working to express.

Period evening gowns are sometimes delightful for you. They express an old-fashioned charm, which is a haunting refrain of your character.

In the house, pretty flowered smocks are fresh and sweet.

46

MAN'S GIRL.—Your personality is a very colourful one already, so be rather constrained about colour in your clothes.

The classic, black frock, trimmed with touches of white, is perhaps your most perfect setting.

Flowers are not really suited to your type, except perhaps a button-hole in a tailored suit.

And beware of any jewellery, which might be described as flashy.

In fact, never wear more than one piece of jewellery at once—the new gilt jewellery would be nice.

Wear hats back off the face to show your charming, friendly smile.

Don't wear too high heels, or furs (except as a trimming) or soft, fluffy materials. Firm, dull, matt surfaces are much better than shiny ones, so avoid satin, ciré or gold or silver tissues.

CLEVER TYPE.—You are not inclined to bother much about clothes. You usually wear them for a long time and like things more for comfort than for effect.

You want to aim at wearing casual clothes, not just any clothes casually.

Loose, rather mannish swagger coats, smart, tailored suits, silk shirts and crisp white blouses, tweeds, hand-knitted sweaters, chamois leather jackets reveal your casual, rather Bohemian nature.

Your country clothes should be chiefly mixture, rather misty shades, like the sea and the sky and the countryside you love so well.

For your town clothes, stick to smooth, firm materials.

If you do not like wearing hats, just don't wear one. You can get away with it. Loose, pull-on tailored felts or hats with large brims if you do wear one.

In the evening you will feel happiest in the classic black velvet gown.

47

PERFECT WIFE.—Deep, rich colours work magic for you. They bring out the warmth of your nature, the spontaneous friendliness and sympathy.

Don't go in for extremes in your clothes. Nothing too feminine, nor too masculine, because you are neither.

Jewels express you better than flowers. The golden brown topaz or jade is lovely.

Wear gaily checked gingham overalls in the house.

Aim at smart simplicity of line with very simple accessories to set off the lovely glowing colours of your clothes.

GOOD TIME GIRL.—You are an exciting person yourself and you want to express this in your clothes without appearing bizarre.

Romantic sleeves, full and caught into little, tight cuffs, skirts with movement in every line, unusual colour contrasts to emphasize your emotional range.

You are the type for amusing accessories, for crazy hats, for the latest American shoes.

In the evening you want to achieve a glamorous effect.

Get a feeling of movement into all your clothes, full, flared skirts, unsweeping hats and big sleeves to express your eager, dynamic self.

CHILDISHLY APPEALING TYPE.—You are the type who looks angelic in breton sailors when you're young and charming and when you're older in off-the-face hats with little fluttery veils.

You can wear the highest of heels and the most impractical of clothes.

Your character is rather fragile and clinging, so don't go in for too strong colours, which belie your personality.

In the evening white is your colour and you look your bewitching self behind a fluttering fan.

And to justify the little minx that you really are, put a drop or two of perfume on the fan before you flutter it !

Flowers are lovely for you.   Wear a cute little posy bang in the front of your hat in the day or fasten your hat under your chin with ribbons, with a tiny posy tucked in the bow.

And wear them in your hair or round your wrists in the evening.

Moss roses, forget-me-nots and primroses or stephanotis are all charming.

GLAMOROUS TYPE.—Your best friend is your tailor.

Simple suits or dresses in black, navy blue or dark brown for daytime in a fairly firm material.

But use touches of white to bring out your romantic streak, such as white ruffles, crisp white pull-on gloves.

Concentrate on sharp, well-defined lines in every single part of your wardrobe—no slurred, blurred contours.

In the evening, bring out your romantic streak in material and colour, but keep the simplicity of design.

You are the type who can wear evening cloaks and capes with a flair.

Avoid fussy, too feminine hats.   Hats with brim and character are right for you.

AN important, in fact an essential, part of Charm is self-confidence. You must be sure of yourself, of the way you look.

A charming woman is always completely sure of herself.   So you must have no doubts in your mind when you go out about your dress.

D

Always spend a minute or two in front of your mirror before you go out. Hold a private pre-view and ask yourself these questions :—

1. Is there anything about me about which I am self-conscious ?

2. Is there anything about me at which I do not want people to look ?

3. Is everything I have on spotlessly clean ?

4. Is everything I have on freshly pressed ?

5. Is everything I have on aired and fresh—no stale cigarette smoke clinging to anything ?

6. Is there anything I have on which is in need of a stitch ?

7. Are the ribbons on my hat frayed at the edges ?

8. Are my gloves and bag and shoes spotlessly clean ?

9. Is there a spotless hanky, faintly perfumed, in my bag ?

10. Is the interior of my bag clean and tidy ?

11. Am I wearing anything, such as flowers, jewellery or an accessory, which would make the finished effect smarter if I took it off ?

12. Does my hat make a perfect frame for the picture of my face ?

13. Am I rightly dressed for the function to which I am going—whether it is to the office or just out shopping for the day's supplies ?

14. Do I look the sort of person I should like to meet myself ?

If there is anything you are not sure about take it off or change it. *Then, when you are sure you are perfect, go out and forget entirely about your appearance.*
You are sure of yourself.
This gives you poise.
And poise is Charm.
At first you will find this little pre-view will take several minutes while you ask yourself these questions and sum yourself up.

50

But, as you get more used to it, it will only need a searching glance into a full-length mirror to send you off confident that you are looking your charming best.

🦎

SET aside one evening each week to spend on your clothes. Go over everything in your wardrobe, press and mend if necessary or send them to be cleaned.

Don't forget to press the ribbons on your hats, to trim them if necessary, and to clean hat linings.

Air the cupboard where you keep your clothes often, and never put anything back in it which smells of cigarette smoke.

Keep your evening clothes and light dresses in special dress bags, which keep out dust.

On each coat hanger, tie a tiny lavender bag. This gives fragrance to everything your wear.

And remember to keep your undies fresh and dainty. No woman can present a really charming exterior if there is the sneaking knowledge at the back of her mind all the time that the underneath is not so good.

Do you ever blush for your undies when you take your frock off in a shop ?

Not for their age, for no one will blame you for that, but because they are crumpled, torn, with a shoulder strap pinned, or not absolutely fresh.

Promise yourself that in future you will never be guilty of these offences, that every day of your life you will be as fresh and dainty as if you were going to a party.

And remember you should never expect stockings to do more than one day of duty.

🦎

ONE part of their wardrobe women often neglect is their nightwear.

They may go out in the daytime looking as fresh and sweet as a daisy, but they slop round the house in a shabby dressing-gown and go to bed in nighties or pyjamas that are but the shadows of their former selves.

"What does it matter when no one sees us?" these women defend themselves.

It does matter. And this is why.

Real charm is a constant thing, not just something put on for parties. It's something you want to be, something you want to live.

Freshness and daintiness at all times is an essential of true charm.

If you go to bed in a pretty nightie, with your curls tied up with a ribbon to match, you will feel unconsciously pleased with yourself and your thoughts will echo your pleasure.

Feeling charming is half way to being charming.

One of the most important garments in your whole wardrobe is your foundation garment. This, even in the cases of the cheapest belt or corset, should be tried on and properly fitted before you buy it.

It is essential that it should fit you like a glove, without a wrinkle, yet it must not constrict your movements or cause discomfort. Brassières must support, not constrict.

Remember that your foundation garment is just that—the FOUNDA-TION. Upon it is built the whole structure.

WHEN adding new additions to your wardrobe, never just "go shopping."

Write down on paper first exactly what you need most, what you want to wear it with and for what occasions you want it.

Then go out and persevere until you find it. Never buy anything on the spur of the moment without first considering its future usefulness.

Don't become flustered in shops and feel that you have to buy "something."

Tell the salesgirl exactly what you are looking for and she will be anxious to help you.

Think of her as someone who is doing her utmost to please you, not as someone who is trying to force you to buy something you don't want.

If you decide there is nothing right for you, tell her so and thank her for her trouble.   Then leave ; don't dither, or she will be forced to continue to try to interest you.

BE YOUR AGE is a very important rule to remember when buying anything.   Never let an outfit make you look absurdly younger or even a little older than you really are.

It is not being true to yourself.   And to be charming, you must be true to yourself.

Never be carried away by a new fashion until you are sure it is right for you, or until you have adapted it to fit in with your general scheme.

There is probably some moderation which is right for you.   You owe it to yourself to discover it !

THE line of your clothes is very important, too.

If you are short you want to wear clothes with long, slim unbroken lines and hats with high brims or crowns to give you height.

But if you are tall, wear shallow crowned hats and wear clothes with basques, belts or sashes on stripes going round the body to break your height.

MOVEMENT

🙠   🙠   🙠

THERE is beauty in lovely movement, there is poetry in a graceful gesture.

One of the loveliest things about youth is the free, flowing, supple movements, but even in old age it is possible to express charm in graceful, dignified movements.

When a girl is seventeen and all the world is so gloriously at her feet, when her muscles are supple willow wands and her bones are pliable and smoothly gliding, when her blood runs fast and urgently in her veins, she is a lovely thing to watch.

Her movements have a breath-taking appeal, she seems to float swiftly and surely through the air. Her feet scarcely touch the ground and all her movements are free.

Watch her running with her hair streaming behind her, every limb moving in perfect rhythm, her head thrown back and her feet flying swiftly and lightly over the ground.

It is this spirit of youth and freedom which you want to keep or recapture in your own movements.

Your step should betray an eagerness for living and the love of life itself.

🙠

STUDY things that are beautiful in movement. Watch trees swaying to and fro in a wind, bending so smoothly and supplely.

Watch swans gliding on a river, arching their long white necks, folding their beautiful, powerful wings.

Watch the deer in a park, stepping so gracefully in and out of the trees, lifting proud heads to each little breeze.

Study the movements and gestures of actresses on the stage, of film stars on the screen, of dancers. Watch the expressive way they move their hands, their necks, the way they carry their heads, how they walk, sit, stand, dance.

Memorize their movements and practise them at home in front of your mirror.

Learn to use your arms and hands in beautifully expressive movements. Don't be afraid to move your arms freely. Practise stretching them above your head when you are alone to get rid of any awkwardness you may have.

Always move your hands from the wrists. Practise circling your hands from the wrists, making little circular gestures.

Try and get this softly, sweeping circular movement from the wrists into your ordinary gestures.

Never thrust something straight at someone or put out your arm straight to pick something up. It is ugly.

But describe a very slight movement with your arm and wrist and it is lovely.

Practise this movement when you are by yourself in your household or office tasks.

At first you will be inclined to exaggerate, but gradually it will become more and more natural and you will find yourself doing it unconsciously.

Practise in front of a mirror, picking things up, handing them to imaginary people, doing all the little homely things you do each day.

HOW do you walk? Smoothly, with a swing, or do you take little, mincing, bobbing steps? Do you place your feet down sole first, one foot in front of the other, keeping the foot straight or do you turn your toes out or in or put your foot down heel first ?

Practise walking round your bedroom. Carry your head well back with your nose in the air !

Don't throw your chest out like a sergeant major, but see that your back is straight and your shoulders aren't sloping or pushing forwards. Take fairly large steps and let your thighs glide past one another. Your knees should brush ever so lightly as you walk.

Let your arms swing freely in time to your body, but don't exaggerate this movement.

Now take the weight out of your feet and walk as though you wanted to get somewhere.

Try walking for at least five minutes each day, concentrating on everything I have told you. Soon you will find you begin to move that way naturally.

A good exercise to practise to make you light footed and to give you good posture is to walk round your room with a book balanced on your head and to pick your feet right off the floor at each step. This helps to give you that gliding movement instead of an ugly jerk. Practise walking round the room on tiptoes barefoot to give you perfect balance.

NOW stand in front of your full-length mirror with your feet together and your hands at your sides. Look at your posture carefully.

Is your head thrown proudly back, giving a clean outline to your throat and chin ?

Is your back absolutely straight and your shoulders square ?

Are your shoulders absolutely dead level ?

When you stand with your legs together, do your knees, shins and ankles touch ?

A good way to test whether you have a straight back is to stand

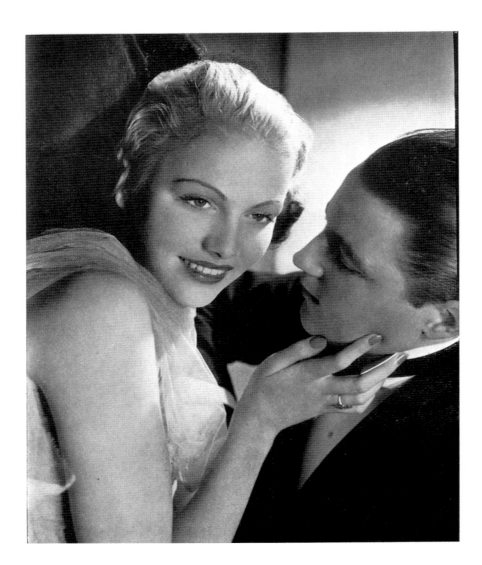

up against a wall with the back of your head and your heels touching the wall. Is the small of your back against the wall? You shouldn't be able to get your hand between the wall and your back.

Are you sure you have no ugly mannerisms when standing?

Do you stand with all your weight on one foot with your hip thrown out of line with your body? Do you twist your legs round one another? Do you droop one shoulder down? Do you poke your head forward? Or stand with your feet apart?

All these little things spoil your stance—and charm.

And how do you sit? Primly on the edge of your chair like the traditional school ma'am or slouched in a chair with your chin on your chest, your legs apart and your skirt above your knees?

There is a saying you can tell whether a woman has breeding by the way she sits.

When you sit down, walk up to the chair squarely, don't sidle up to it. Turn on your toes and sit down. Once seated, don't scrape your chair or move it about nervously feeling if your dress is smooth under you.

Smooth your dress with your hands when you first sit down and make sure it is not showing your knees, then forget about it. Hold your head up and keep your back straight, but don't be stiff. Let your hands lie relaxed in your lap or on the arms of the chair, but don't fiddle with things. Hands are lovely in repose, but can be very irritating when they fidget.

Keep your legs and feet together or cross your feet if you feel more comfortable that way.

Place a chair in front of your mirror and practise sitting. You will then know just how it looks to others.

MOST women look ugly when they run—watch the average woman, in the street running for a 'bus. She takes little, short, stilted steps.

She holds herself stiffly and gracelessly, she frowns as if it is an extreme discomfort and she clutches her parcels or bag to her and wobbles in the most ungainly way.

You should be able to run just as freely and gracefully as you walk. Practise it some time when you are alone in the garden or in a park at a moment when no one is looking.   After all, you can always pretend you are in a hurry !

Don't sink down on your feet at each step, just touch the ground with the soles of your feet.   Run as lightly as possible and lean forward when you run, in a graceful line.

Hold your head up and lift your face to the wind.   Hold your arms naturally at your side and take long swinging steps.   Keep the picture of that lovely young girl running that I described in the beginning of this lesson in your mind as you run.

I CANNOT overstress the importance of keeping your body young and elastic.

Of course, as you get older, you are bound to lose some of the suppleness of youth, but your movements take on a new dignified graciousness and charm—if you let them.

But you can still keep some of its elasticity.

Walking or dancing are both excellent for keeping your body supple. If you don't get the chance to do much of either, do a little skipping or a few exercises each morning before breakfast.

Take some outdoor exercise regularly each week.   Tennis, swimming, or rowing in the summer, and riding, golf or bicycling in the winter.

Skating, either ice or roller skating, is good, too.

Tap dancing is very good exercise, too, and in most of the big towns there are classes several nights a week, which you can attend very cheaply.

IT is impossible to keep your body supple and graceful if you allow it to get fat.

You should watch your weight carefully and weigh yourself at least once a week. Any great increase in weight should be immediately counteracted by diet, exercise, massage or special baths.

The correct average weights should be as follows for women of various heights and ages :

Height ft. in.	Age 15-19 st. lb.	Age 20-24 st. lb.	Age 25-29 st. lb.	Age 30-34 st. lb.	Age 35-40 st. lb.
4 11	7 12	8 1	8 4	8 7	8 10
5 0	8 0	8 3	8 6	8 9	8 12
5 1	8 2	8 5	8 8	8 11	9 0
5 2	8 5	8 8	8 10	8 13	9 3
5 3	8 8	8 11	8 13	9 2	9 6
5 4	8 11	9 0	9 3	9 6	9 10
5 5	9 0	9 3	9 6	9 10	10 0
5 6	9 4	9 7	9 10	10 0	10 4
5 7	9 8	9 11	10 0	10 4	10 8
5 8	9 12	10 1	10 4	10 8	10 12
5 9	10 1	10 5	10 8	10 12	11 2
5 10	10 5	10 9	10 12	11 1	11 5

Add on 3 lb. for every five years over forty up to sixty.

You should not be heavier than this, but don't worry if you are lighter as long as you keep a steady average and don't lose weight.

It is wise, too, to check your measurements on the average every three months, so that you can beware of any slight thickening and counteract it.

HOW TO FIND FRIENDS

THE woman who has no friends does not live her life to the full.

One is not meant to be alone. The contact and companionship with one's fellow beings is necessary to everyone.

If you are too much alone, you dwell in too narrow a world, and you become too introspective.

Are you lonely? Do you long for friends and yet not know how to make them?

Have you never known the joy of walking in the country with the rain and wind on your face with a friend beside you?

Have you never known the fun of talking with a friend by the firelight?

Have you never known the triumph of friends who have stood by you in trouble?

Have you never known the privilege of helping a friend in trouble?

Some women seem to have the gift of friendship. They keep their friends for ever, wherever they go they establish contacts and sympathies with others.

Their friendship is valued by others and they seem to draw others as moths fly to a light.

LET us discover first if you have the qualities of friendship.

I have drawn up a questionnaire for you to fill in. I want you to

60

think about each question carefully and answer it very honestly either
"yes" or "no", on the dotted line opposite the questions.

1. Can you say that you never discuss the failings of
one of your friends with another ?   . . . .

2. Do you always stand up for an absent friend when
you hear them spoken of disparagingly in your presence ?   . . . .

3. Are you always ready to give up your time to help
a friend ?   . . . .

4. Have you always stood by your friends in trouble ?. . . . .

5. Can you say that you never impose on friendships
by pouring out your grievances and troubles ?   . . . .

6. Can you say that you never lie to your friends or
make excuses instead of always telling them the truth
kindly and tactfully ?   . . . .

7. Would you go out of your way to do something
kind for a friend ?   . . . .

8. If a friend is ill or goes abroad, do you let her know
you are thinking about her ?   . . . .

9. Are you always ready to share what you have of the
world's goods with a friend who has struck a patch of
misfortune ?   . . . .

10. Can you say that you are never envious of anything your friends possess ?   . . . .

11. Can you say that you are never suspicious of your
friends' actions and motives ?   . . . .

12. Can you say that you never cancel an appointment
with a friend if something more interesting turns up,
unless you include her in it ?   . . . .

13. Do you never break your word to a friend? . . . .

14. If a friend gives you her confidence, do you *always* keep it strictly to yourself? . . . .

15. If a friend lets you down, do you never abuse her to others for her ingratitude? . . . .

16. Are you always ready to help her bring out the charm that is in her? . . . .

17. Can you say that you are never a little bit jealous if you introduce two of your friends and they strike up a great friendship? . . . .

18. If you know your friend is doing something dis-honourable, do you tell her frankly and nicely that you feel she is letting herself down, but do not withdraw your friendship if she ignores your advice? . . . .

19. If you hear something to a friend's discredit, do you ask her about it openly and frankly before believing it and give her a chance to defend herself? . . . .

20. Can you say that you never abuse a friendship by clinging to the other person or becoming maudlinly sentimental about them? . . . .

Now count up the numbers of times you have answered "Yes". If your score is 20 you are the perfect friend. If your score is between 15 and 20 you are capable of great friendship. If your score is between 10 and 15 you have an average capacity for friendship. But if your score is below 10, there is something wrong in your attitude to other people and you must alter this before you can find true and lasting friendship.

And if your score is below 5, it reveals that you are selfish and far too self-centred and you must work hard to become unselfish and think of others before yourself. No one should rest content until they can honestly score at least 15.

Take all the points to which you have answered "No" and work at them with determination.

Only *you* can alter these things in yourself. And if you do, you will be a far happier person.

PERSONALITY has a lot to do with attracting friendship. Women with no personality or ideas seldom have many friends.

The more you learn to express your personality and put it over, the more you will have for others, the more they will prize your company. If you want to make friends make yourself as interesting a person as you possibly can. Read, travel, play games, have hobbies, go to films, plays, lectures, art galleries, museums.

Join a club where they specialize in whatever you are interested in.

Take your holidays in one of the many conducted parties.

If you live alone, why not live in a club or hotel for a while and you will soon get to know people ? If you want to learn to speak a foreign language or some special craft or knowledge or business training, why not attend evening classes? This is especially good for young people as you're bound to meet heaps of other youngsters of both sexes.

Another good source is amateur dramatics. In almost every town or village there is a dramatic society. You will find them great fun and they certainly do break the ice.

Meet as many and as varied people as you can, then you will have more to choose your friends from. As a general rule it is better to choose your friends from your own social equals. You will have more in common this way and will be more at ease with each other.

WHEN you have made a contact there are several important things to remember.

Never try to force a friendship by overdoing one's advances. If you do this, anyone with an inner wall of reserve will instinctively withdraw.

Never wear a friendship out in the beginning by overuse. If you're always seeing the same person, always doing things with them, writing to them, telephoning them, talking to them, the friendship soon gets stale and you find yourself quietly dropped.

Never make the mistake of trying to make too many friends. In friendship it is quality and not quantity that counts. If you have a few good staunch friends you can count yourself far luckier than the woman who has dozens of flighty passing acquaintances. And remember that other people are probably just as ready to make friends as you are. So never hesitate to make the first advances. If you meet someone you like instinctively, who immediately appeals to you, suggest you meet again.

And if you feel shy think that the other person is probably shy too and concentrate on setting her at ease. In your efforts to make her forget her shyness, you will find yours has disappeared. Go through life ready to make friends. *Expect* the loveliest things from life. *Expect* to meet the loveliest, most interesting people.

Each new person you meet, think of their potentialities. *Expect* the best from them, but do not deceive yourself if you do not get it.

If the person is not nice, if you feel that they are not worthy of your friendship, do not offer it. Friendship should be an uplifting thing, something that calls forth the best in one.

Keep this air of expectation in your life, in your thoughts and on your face.

Look as if each new person you meet may be the nicest person you've ever met.

Look as if each party you go to is going to be greater fun than any party you've ever been to.

This air of expectancy gives your face a charming vivacity and draws people to you.

They subconsciously want to fulfil your expectations and so it brings out the best that is in others.

ALWAYS be kind and sweet to everybody you meet—friends, acquaintances, servants, officials, fellow workers, travellers.

Never let yourself down by being rude or impatient.

At the end of each day, go over all the contacts you have made in your mind. Were you as nice to every person you met as you might have been?

Is there anything you might have done for anyone that you didn't do?

Start from the beginning of the day. And don't forget anyone you may have met casually, someone in a bus or a train, or the office.

Did you leave anyone with the slightest feeling of resentment?

Ask yourself honestly if you tried to be *charming* to every single person you met.

AS you become slowly a much happier, freer, fuller, more charming person, beware of becoming critical of others who have not learnt to develop their inherent charm and personalities in the same way.

Always be tolerant of others and considerate of their feelings.

The charming woman has a perfect sense of tact.

She always knows instinctively what to say and *what not to say*.

The woman who believes in "speaking her mind" or "calling a spade a spade" is never charming. She is one of two things, either painfully self-conscious with a colossal feeling of inferiority—hence the need for bluff frankness—or a fool.

E   65

You must cultivate a charming sense of tact.
Remember these six rules and never, never break them.

1. Never make a joke or wise-crack at someone else's expense.
2. If someone asks you a question which you feel it would be kinder not to answer frankly, evade it without telling a lie.

   For example, if a friend introduces you to her fiancé whom you do not like and she asks you afterwards what you think of him, say something that will please her and yet relieve you of the necessity of answering her question, such as "He's a very lucky man" or "I'm sure you'll both be very happy." Or praise something about him that you really think is admirable.
3. If someone has just experienced something unpleasant or a great sorrow, be careful that you don't remind them of it either in your words or, more important, in the manner you talk to them. People have a maddening way of talking to someone who has just been bereaved in a sort of hushed, shocked whisper. Be natural at all times in your manner.
4. Never make anyone feel hurt, angry, indignant or embarrassed by anything you may say or do either deliberately or thoughtlessly.

   Remember, you want to bring more happiness and beauty to others as well as yourself.
5. If someone unwittingly or perhaps even knowingly, offends another person in your presence, don't be paralysed by it. Jump into the gap at once with a new idea, something that will take both their minds off the subject.
6. Let people know that they can trust you, never betray a confidence, never let people down. Never betray someone else to another person. Don't gossip maliciously and don't pry into other people's affairs. The charm of being able to mind one's own business is a great one.

66

CONVERSATION

OFTEN the plainest woman in a room receives the most attention from both men and women. Charm is her secret. The charm of a sympathetic nature, of a genuine interest in others. The charm of being a good listener but capable of good conversation when the occasion arises.

She is always completely at ease with others and knows how to make the other person feel at ease with her. This trait of inspiring those with whom she comes in contact with self-confidence endears her to everyone she meets.

You know yourself how you blossom out and think of all sorts of amusing and interesting things you have to say when you feel someone is genuinely interested in your opinions.

Always be ready to be interested when you meet a rather dull-looking woman. Don't think: "My goodness, what a bore, how can I get away?" and let your eyes go roaming around the room looking for someone who appears more interesting. Instead think: "Here is someone new, someone who has all sorts of interesting and exciting possibilities. I must set her at ease and bring out the best that is in her."

Greet her as if you were really pleased to meet her. And keep your eyes on her face all the time you are talking with her. Don't stare blankly, your eyes never wavering. Let your face talk and listen with you, smiling a little, sometimes changing its expression with your thoughts.

OF course, it's quite impossible to put anyone at their ease if you are nervous and shy yourself. Stop thinking about your own nervousness. Stop thinking about yourself altogether.

Think of the other person all the time. As long as you are giving mentally you will not feel shy or nervous.

Some of us suffer from an uncertainty of what to talk about. It is no use whatever being a good listener if the other person has nothing to talk about.

You must be able to take the lead swiftly and surely if need be.

Not everyone can be a witty and amusing conversationalist, but every woman can have a fund of interesting and varied conversation.

Keep yourself well informed about the world's affairs, by reading a newspaper thoroughly every day and perhaps one of the news magazines. This alone will give you an unfailing supply of subjects to talk about.

If you have a hobby such as gardening, collecting something or making your own clothes—talk about it, don't be afraid of boring other people. Everyone likes to hear someone talking about something that really interests them.

The same thing applies to your job or the game you play.

But don't dwell on one subject too long. When you have said all there is to say, switch to something else.

IT is a charming trait to try and find a link in your conversation. A consecutive line of thought is more pleasing than a series of stops and starts. For instance, suppose you have been talking about gardening, you have compared notes on your respective gardens and you feel that the conversation will shortly start to drag a little. One of you has just been describing the wonderful bed of peonies she had last summer. Say brightly and expectantly as if the memory really excited you : "Oh did you see Epstein's flower painting of the peonies? I shall never forget the colour of them and the richness of the blooms; I could almost smell their perfume as I looked at them."

The other person mayn't have seen any of his flower paintings and say so, but may mention they have seen one or two of his bronze heads or busts.

There you have another topic for conversation at once. You can mention the ones you have seen too, what you thought of them and where you saw them. If it was in a museum, you can go on to some other exhibits in the museum, if it was abroad you can discuss that country and so on.

It is an excellent thing to practise this train of thought, as nothing keeps the ball rolling as effectively in a conversation.

You may say : "That's all very well, I can usually get on all right once I get started, but *how* do I start ?"

This depends very much, of course, on where you are and who it is you are meeting. Suppose, for instance, you have just arrived at a cocktail party, have greeted your hostess, who has probably introduced you to a young man or woman. A good opening is to be amusingly frank. Say exactly what you are thinking at the moment. "Thank heavens, I'm really inside at last, I always suffer agonies of shyness when I walk up the steps. Do you ever feel like that ?"

Or "Isn't Vi (the hostess) perfectly charming ? Do you know her well ?" or "What a lovely party it looks; I always adore Vi's cocktail parties. Have you been to any before ?" If it is a smartly-dressed woman with something about her you particularly admire say : "I simply adore your hat. I saw it the moment I came into the room; wherever did you find it ?" She will be pleased with your genuine praise and your conversation will turn on hats for those first few minutes.

But supposing it is a little group of people you have been introduced to and they have been discussing something which they broke off when you arrived.

Say brightly : "Do go on. What is the subject under debate ?" Someone will probably say : "We were just discussing . . ." Then say : "I'm afraid I know nothing about . . . but I'd love to learn," if you do know nothing about it.

But if you are interested say so : "Oh how lovely, I'm so interested in . . ."

That makes you part of the little group at once and has done away with the necessity for them abandoning their conversation in order to start something which includes you.

Now supposing you find yourself seated between two strangers at a luncheon or dinner.

Neither seems disposed to break the ice, perhaps one is very nervous, revealing this by twiddling with his tie or clearing his throat rather noisily as if he were about to make a speech. Turn to him with a charming smile and say : "I believe you're just as nervous as I am. These formal affairs always terrify me, don't they you ?"

This will disarm him completely, the personal touch will set him at ease and unless he is a very dull person he will make the next move.

If you want to draw both men into a conversation at once a good beginning is to smile wickedly at them both and say : "Well, who's going to make the first conversational effort ?"

But if you feel these are too flippant openings for the partners you are confronted with, try something very general like : "I'm longing to peep at the menu, do you think you could rescue one for me ?" Food is always a safe subject as most people are interested in that. It's amazing how people thaw when the subject of food is mentioned.

MAKE certain you have no annoying conversational habits which make you appear unnatural, affected, or, still worse, a bore.
Ask yourself these questions out loud.

(1) When I think of something amusing to say do I become so obsessed with it that I break in while the other person is talking ?

(2) Have I any pet words which appear time and time again in my conversation ?

(3) Do I sometimes say "um" when listening to someone instead of yes ?

(4) Have I any hangovers from my schoolgirl slang in my conversation, such as "coo—", "crumbs", "crikey", and so on ?

(5) When I am listening to someone, am I quite sure that my mouth is never open ?

(6) Am I ever guilty of monopolizing the conversation, not giving anyone else a chance to get a word in ?

(7) Do I talk in clichés ?

(8) If I use slang, am I sure the words I use never jar on the feelings of others ?

(9) Do I ever adopt a rather la-di-da tone and conversation when talking to someone who is my social superior ?

(10) Am I ever guilty of pouring out my grievances to strangers ?

(11) If I wise-crack am I ever guilty of doing it at the expense of others ?

(12) Am I ever guilty of discussing one person with another in disparaging terms ?

The more you do, the more you think about and the more you read, the more you will have to talk about and the more interesting you are to other people.

71

It mayn't be possible for everyone to travel, but everyone can read about foreign parts and travel in their thoughts with a book.

Go to as many new films and plays as you can and read the critics' opinions on them afterwards to compare with your own.

Visit art galleries and museums, old buildings and churches, and attend lectures on any subject you are interested in.

Learn to travel in your thoughts. Say to yourself: "I want to travel, travel, travel. In my thoughts, in my deeds, in the words I read." Keep your mind supplied with new and interesting things to think about.

Read the latest books. It's so easy to be well read nowadays when you can borrow a book for 2d. a week from one of the many good libraries.

THERE are a certain number of books, which every woman who would like to consider herself well-read should read. Make up your mind to read one each week in the next year. Nothing broadens your mind so much as good reading.

THERE is no better way of improving your knowledge of the English language than reading. You will learn new words, new phrases, new sentence constructions.

If you feel that your vocabulary is rather deficient and you would like to enlarge it a little, learn one new word from your dictionary each day and practise introducing them into your conversation.

I have picked these books to give you as varied reading as possible.

Great Expectations—Charles Dickens.
William Shakespeare's Collected Plays.
Rob Roy—Sir Walter Scott.

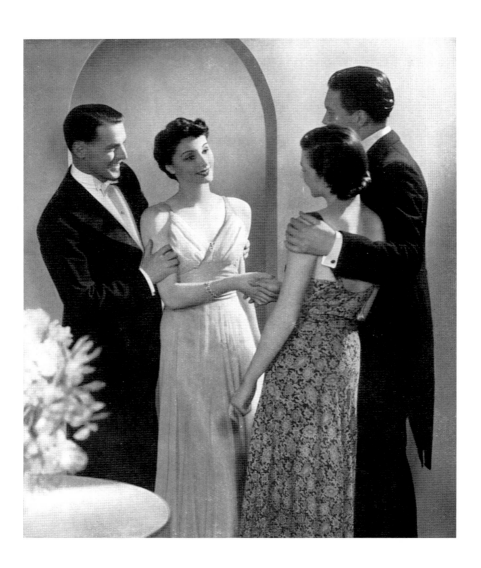

Vanity Fair—Thackeray.
The Vicar of Wakefield—Oliver Goldsmith.
Pride and Prejudice—Jane Austen.
Wuthering Heights—Emily Brontë.
Jane Eyre—Charlotte Brontë.
Charlotte Brontë—Mrs. Gaskell.
Tess of the D'Urbervilles—Thomas Hardy.
Richard Feverel—George Meredith.
Monte Cristo—Alexandre Dumas.
Gulliver's Travels—Swift.
Barchester Towers—Trollope.
To the Lighthouse—Woolf.
The Importance of Being Earnest—Oscar Wilde.
Sheridan's Plays.
Ghosts—Ibsen.
Anna Karenina—Tolstoy.
Faust—Goethe.
Madame Bovary—Flaubert.
Père Goriot—Balzac.
Don Quixote—Cervantes.
Forsyte Saga—John Galsworthy.
Sentimental Tommy—J. M. Barrie.
Man and Superman—George Bernard Shaw.
An Outline of History—H. G. Wells.
Art Through the Ages—Helen Gardner.
Van Loon's Geography—Hendrik van Loon.
The Mysterious Universe—James Jeans.
Experiment with Time—James Dunne.
Dewer Rides—L. A. G. Strong.
Alice in Wonderland—Lewis Carroll.
Kim—Rudyard Kipling.
Treasure Island—R. L. Stevenson.

Inside Europe—John Gunther.
The Path to Rome—Hilaire Belloc.
O. Henry's Short Stories.
Waste Land—T. S. Eliot.
Arabian Nights.
Green Apple Harvest—Sheila Kaye-Smith.
The Purple Land—W. H. Hudson
Pilgrim's Progress—John Bunyan.
W. B. Yeats's Collected Poems.
Dante (Carey's translation).
The Flying Inn—G. K. Chesterton.

AND now I want us to consider your voice. For no matter how interesting and amusing your conversation, a displeasing voice can make people not want to listen to you. Your voice should be pitched low and you should speak slowly and clearly, pronouncing all the syllables clearly.

If it is at all possible have a record made of your speaking voice. You can have it done very cheaply and it is invaluable, for giving you an idea of how your voice sounds to others. You never catch the true tones of it when listening to it yourself in the ordinary way.

Listen to its timing, its cadence, its pronunciation, its tone. Most voices would be much more attractive if they were lower.

It is quite easy to deepen your voice. Stop talking at the top of your head or at the top of your lungs.

Correct breathing does a lot towards improving your voice. You should practise breathing down deep as they used to make you do in your singing lessons at school.

Speak a short phrase such as "Day is Done" in your ordinary voice. Now repeat it, sinking it a tone lower in your throat. Now repeat it again another tone lower.

Do it as deep as you can without straining your voice at all. Practise this each day with different words and phrases. Remember to sink your voice when you speak. If at first you do it consciously, it will soon become unconscious.

Think of any voice you admire on the stage, on the radio, or perhaps that of a friend or acquaintance. They are all deeply pitched.

There is something thrilling about a deep rich voice in a woman. Don't overdo it and make your voice sound unnatural and don't try and copy somebody else's voice.

That is *their* voice. You want to make *your own* more beautiful. And you can do this by finding the most attractive pitch and making it your normal speaking voice.

Beware of a Garbo throatiness unless you are sure it suits your personality and whatever you do don't let a nasal pitch spoil the charm of your voice.

A man said to me once of a mutual friend of ours : "I could listen to X for hours, she talks such utter rubbish but in such a beautiful voice."

When you have successfully deepened your voice, get a caressive, soft quality into it.

Make even the most commonplace phrases sound exciting and romantic. Repeat a lovely phrase such as : "Soft moonlight"; "I love you"; "A cluster of pearls" out loud, lingering over the words lovingly. Now repeat a more ordinary phrase such as "How do you do", or "I'm so glad you could come", keeping the same tone of voice. You will be amazed at the charm of your own voice.

LOOKING BACK—AND FORWARD

$\mathscr{L}$ $\mathscr{L}$ $\mathscr{L}$

CHARM—"Oh, it's—it's—sort of a bloom on a woman . . ." these are other lovely words Sir James Barrie used when writing of charm.

It seems to describe so perfectly all the sweetness, the grace, the poise, the shining love of life that makes for charm in a woman.

We have already come a long way together on this road that leads to charm, but there is still a long way to go.

And when we say good-bye at the end, when you go forth alone into the world with all your new-found knowledge, I hope that I shall have helped you to find this sweetness, this grace, this poise, this love of life, this bloom.

Already you should feel a happier, freer person, more at peace with yourself and with the whole world, more self-confident.

We have talked together on many subjects. Let us go over them briefly together.

Remember how we talked of your attitude to yourself and your attitude to others.

Of the faults that might be spoiling your chances of charm and how to dispel them.

Of the necessity of keeping yourself and everything around you dainty and charming.

Of serenity and how to achieve it.

Then we spoke of the importance of learning to know yourself, of discovering your glandular theme type and developing the best that is in you.

76

Of the use of clothes and colour to emphasize your personality.

Of the importance of keeping your clothes exquisite.

Of the use of cosmetics and beauty aids to enhance the natural beauty of your face and body.

Of the importance of good health.

We decided to keep something beautiful always near us to inspire our thoughts with beauty.

We talked of beautiful movements, lovely gestures and the importance of keeping the body youthful and supple.

And then in the last lesson we discussed your voice. How you can make it more beautiful to the ear. How to be a good listener and how to acquire a fund of interesting and varied conversation and express it.

AND now we are going on together triumphantly to the end of this course.

We have found the magic key together, but we still have to learn how to use it.

How to use it to open the doors of love and happiness, and having found them, how to keep them in your life.

We are going to talk about etiquette together, not only the conversational rules of society, but how to turn them to charming account for yourself.

We are going to bring beauty into your home and learn how to make your home a perfect setting for you, not just a place where you eat and sleep.

And finally we are going to discuss the enemies of charm, times in a woman's life when it is particularly difficult to express the charm that is in her soul.

So let us go on together with joy and determination in our hearts.

ARE you sure you are applying everything you have learnt so far in your own home among your family as well as to the outside world?

If you keep your most charming side just for your friends and acquaintances whom you meet outside your home, you are not being true to yourself.

It is like keeping a best dress for Sundays only. And the smart, charming woman doesn't have Sunday clothes any more. She looks her charming best all, and every, day.

Real charm is like this too. It is always there. It does not switch on and off like a tap.

So practise all the things you've learned *all the time*, both inside and outside your home.

NOW I want you to sit in front of your mirror, think of something pleasant, and smile.

Do this several times in different ways.

Imagine you are meeting someone and give a welcoming smile.

Pretend someone has said something funny and give an amused little smile.

Think of something sweet that someone has said to you and give a tender smile.

Pretend someone has just told you a very tall story and give a mocking little smile.

Imagine that you are very sad and someone says something cheering to you and give a wistful smile.

Think of someone who has done something kind for you and give a grateful smile.

Imagine you see somebody across the room, obviously left out of things and feeling rather shy and self-conscious, and send them a friendly, cheering smile.

Watch your face all the time.

Does your smile express your moods?

It should do. A face that has vivacity is charming to watch.

Pretend you are a film star and have to portray all these emotions on the screen.

Practise them in front of your mirror until they feel natural.

Does your smile include your eyes? A smile if it leaves out the eyes never realizes its full charm.

Make your smile a lovely thing to see, make it express your delight in the world. Make it a password to other peoples' affection.

Beware of letting your smile become an affected smile by too much practising.

You must always smile from within—from the soul.

The more you smile, the softer and sweeter your face will become.

There is a little exercise I always practise myself when I feel my face is looking strained, tired, or just blank.

I "think," a little smile. It does wonderful things to the sensitive tiny muscles round your mouth. Try it yourself. I always do this last thing every night before I close my eyes to go to sleep. I relax all over and "think" a little smile.

Make a resolution to do this every night of your life. It sends you to sleep with your face relaxed and a sweet expression playing round your mouth.

THERE is one other kind of smile that is important, the deepening smile that breaks into laughter.

Too sudden laughter, without the softening influence of the smile is not often attractive. It should be like throwing a pebble into a pool, sending out soft, little ripples, wider and wider until they cover the whole pond.

Is your laughter sweet to hear? Or does it, like your voice, need deepening? Practise deepening its pitch just as you did your voice.

Remember that soft laughter is much more attractive than loud laughter.

If you are inclined to giggle when you get nervous, you must exert every scrap of self-control to stop it.

Not only is it an ugly and irritating habit, but it admits that you haven't the perfect self-control of the charming woman.

People remember laughter as they remember your smile and you must make them both equally fragrant memories.

One very important thing to remember is that you can't smile too often, but you can laugh too often. Too frequent laughter becomes irritating, monotonous and meaningless.

But a smile has as many moods as your face and never tires.

W E are not all born with a sense of humour, but there is no doubt that it can be cultivated.

It is an invaluable weapon to possess against all the cares and worries and little tragedies of everyday life.

It is a grand thing to be able to see the funny side of things, and laugh even when the joke is against you.

A sense of humour makes you wonderfully easy to live with and endears you to your friends.

Men especially adore a woman with a sense of humour and you can bring no greater gift to a marriage.

Learn to laugh at life and yourself as well as others.

Develop a tolerance and friendliness towards humanity.

And *never grouse* if something is wrong or someone is imposing upon you. Say so frankly and try to put it right but don't grumble about it to others.

They have little troubles of their own and want to be cheered by your presence, not further depressed.

Never inflict your own worries on others unless they have a right to know.

And never listen to other people's confidential grumbles either.

This is very important as they are invariably just letting off steam to you and hate you afterwards for knowing these too intimate things about their life, their home and their friends.

Their instinctive reaction will be to avoid you in the future and you will lose their friendship.

Always try to switch the conversation into more impersonal channels as soon as someone begins to get over-confidential.

Then if they persist, say that you think it useless to discuss the matter with you as you do not feel competent to advise them.

Do not be at all smug and don't let them feel snubbed or they will be hurt and antagonistic.

Build up a little wall of reserve inside yourself beyond which no one can go, a sense of the preciousness of your own soul.

Never let this inner self down. Always live up to the highest and the best that is in you.

This inner wall of reserve some people call mystery.

This mysteriousness rouses people's interest. They want to know what lies behind it. It gives you that thing called glamour.

A man once said to me : "I have been married to my wife for twenty years and I still think she's the most charming and the most mysterious woman in the world."

What a lovely compliment for a husband of twenty years !

I knew his wife. She was rather plain to look at, rather fat and she dressed very badly.

But she had the most charming expression, a lovely low, caressing voice and this elusive quality of mystery. I was not surprised that her husband was still her devoted lover after all that time.

WHEN I think of her now I always remember the haunting fragrance of the perfume she used. It expressed her personality so beautifully.

It's funny how the memory of a perfume stays with one, especially if it expresses the personality of its wearer.

I have a friend who is tall and willowy with small fragile features, cloudy black hair and a rather languorous disposition, and a skin like magnolia petals.

Whenever I think of her I smell gardenias very faintly. She always uses Chanel's gardenia perfume and it suits her personality so beautifully, that it has become part of the memory she leaves behind.

Does your perfume do this for you? Is it so much part of you that people have only to smell it to remember you?

It is much better to discover a perfume that is the perfect expression of your personality and then use it consistently.

Otherwise the memory becomes confused and blurred.

It is much more economic to put your perfume on with a spray, and it distributes the scent more evenly. Spray it round your throat and hair and behind your ears. But don't put it on your dresses or furs as even the best perfume may go stale or stain.

PERFUME is so exquisitely important. A woman without perfume is like a flower without a scent.

But it must be just right, it must express her moods, her personality, her way of life.

HOW TO FIND *LOVE*

"All thoughts, all passions, all delights,
Whatever stirs this mortal frame,
All are but ministers of Love,
And feed his sacred flame."—(COLERIDGE).

LOVE is the most beautiful thing in the world. It is also the strongest emotion.

It has triumphed above hate, fear, evil, patriotism, religion, and human ties and conventions.

It has transformed men into gods ; it has turned women into angels.

A woman in love has truly entered into her kingdom.

YOU now know that there is no need to be lonely. You have learnt the art of friendship, you have made new friends.

But no woman is truly happy unless she has love in her life.

Every woman has the power to make some man happy and contented and glad to be alive.

In your two little hands and in your heart lies the power to make a man's life hell or a little paradise on earth.

"A guardian angel o'er his life presiding,
Doubling his pleasures, and his cares dividing."

Those two lines of Samuel Rogers' hold for me a lovely definition of wifehood in its highest sense.

If you are married I want you to ask yourself this question out loud and think well and deeply before you reply in your heart : "How much joy and beauty do I bring to my marriage ? Can I say that . . . is truly happy in his union with me ?"

This is such a difficult question to answer that I have decided to enlarge upon it.

Women are less inclined to be honest with themselves over love than over any other subject.

They deliberately shut their eyes and wilfully believe that everything is perfect when, in reality, love is slipping away from their grasp.

This refusal to recognize facts and to do something about it before it is too late is often the cause of great heartbreak.

When a husband suddenly seeks fresh fields, it is usually not because he is particularly fickle or because the other woman is younger or prettier, but because the wife has been stupidly blind about causes and reactions.

This can happen to any woman, because it is a natural feminine instinct to disregard blindly any imperfections in her love.

For a really happy marriage, for a perfect marriage, it is essential to face facts and to be terribly honest with oneself.

I believe that if every woman would take stock of her marriage four times a year, as they do in big and important businesses, it would open her eyes, warn her if necessary and make her union a hundred times happier.

I have drawn up a questionnaire to help you.

Do not look upon it as a game. It is not. It has been drawn up as a sort of insurance policy that you will not take love for granted.

For love should never become a monotonous, hum-drum existence. It is a vital, living thing like a beautiful plant.

If you tend it carefully and set it in the sunshine, and water it regularly, it will grow strong and beautiful.

84

But if you leave it in some dark little corner, with no water or sunshine and let weeds grow round it, it will slowly wither up and die.

And once it is dead, it seldom comes to life again.

*N*OW *ask yourself these questions.   Think about each one carefully and answer it very honestly, either "Yes" or "No" on the dotted line opposite the question.*

1. Am I content with my husband as a mate ? . . . . . .
2. Do I let him know that I am content with him ? . . . . . .
3. Can I say that I never grumble about our lack of this world's goods or fret for things he is unable to provide ? . . . . . .
4. Do we discuss money matters openly and sympathetically together ? . . . . . .
5. Can I say that I never nag him in front of other people ?. . . . . .
6. Can I say that I never nag him when we are alone ? . . . . . .
7. Do I believe in my heart that he always tells me the truth ? . . . . . .
8. Can I say that there is no subject he hesitates to discuss with me because of disagreement or my disapproval ? . . . . . .
9. Does he talk to me about his work ? . . . . . .
10. Can I say that I never discuss his failings with others in front of him ? . . . . . .
11. Can I say that I never discuss his failings with others behind his back ? . . . . . .
12. Am I sympathetic about his weaknesses and failings ? . . . . . .
13. Am I always absolutely honest with him ? . . . . . .
14. Is there a perfect feeling of trust between us ? . . . . . .

15. Can I say that I am never suspicious of his movements ? . . . . . .
16. Do I ever tell him I love him ? . . . . . .
17. Do I ever show him I love him by my actions ? . . . . . .
18. Do I ever look at him as if I loved him ? . . . . . .
19. Do I ever flirt with him a little ? . . . . . .
20. Do I join whole-heartedly with him in our sexual love ? . . . . . .
21. Is there perfect sympathy and understanding between us about sexual life ? . . . . . .
22. Do I praise him when he merits it ? . . . . . .
23. Does he ever pay me compliments ? . . . . . .
24. Is there lots of laughter and fun in our household ? . . . . . .
25. Can I say that I never use tears to get my own way ? . . . . . .
26. Do I tease him lovingly into doing things instead of nagging at him ? . . . . . .
27. Do I show him that I'm pleased to see him when he gets home in the evenings ? . . . . . .
28. Can I say that he never gets pushed into the background by my children's demands ? . . . . . .
29. Do I treat the children as a communal blessing and encourage him to take an interest in, and help with, them ? . . . . . .
30. Do I let him know that he is more important to me than anything else in the world ? . . . . . .

Now add up all the times you answered "Yes". If it is thirty times, you are a perfect wife!

If you score between twenty-five and twenty-nine, he is a lucky man.

If you score between twenty and twenty-four, you are an excellent wife.

If it is between fifteen and nineteen, you are an averagely good wife.

Below fourteen is rather below average and shows that you need to take yourself in hand.

If it is below nine you are a bad wife, so open your eyes and do something about it before it is too late.

And if your score is below four, then you're giving your poor husband a very bad deal, and if he hasn't left you already, he soon will !

No one should be content until they can attain a score of at least twenty.

Look at all the questions to which you answered "No" and determine to do something about them.

Keep this list of questions carefully and ask yourself again in about three months' time.

RELATIVES and friends are often a great cause of disagreement in marriage and more than one home I know of has been broken up by interfering in-laws.

You do not want to cheapen yourself by jealousy or bickering.

You must avoid all discord in your beautiful new life.

Never antagonize your husband over any of his friends and relatives or say anything disparaging about them in his presence.

Be pleasant to them always when you meet, but avoid them as much as possible if you really dislike them.

Don't try to stop him seeing them, because he probably won't, and it only belittles you in his eyes.

If it is your friends or relatives who are causing the trouble, just arrange things so that they come to the house when he is out or you meet them outside.

Always tell him you are going to see them though, so that he does not feel you are keeping anything from him.

NEVER discuss your husband or your relationship with him with anyone, except perhaps with a doctor or a priest if you need advice.

The tie between you is a precious, secret thing and should be treated as such.

Never let any little thing appear too much effort to keep your marriage bright and beautiful.

Keep your body just as slim and fresh and beautiful after marriage as before.

Be even more fastidious and careful about cleanliness and sweetness and always try to look beautiful for your husband.

Pretty flowered overalls or house coats, a touch of lipstick, and hair shining from the hairbrush and a smiling face at the breakfast table leave a pleasant memory all day.

And to come home at night and find your wife looking as if she had been dressing up specially for him—well, what husband could not help but be flattered?

Be charmingly fastidious about your actions and belongings if you share a room. Keep all your little, personal toilet things out of his sight.

I don't mean by this that you should powder your nose always in the bathroom!

I think men like to watch their wives making-up their faces as long as it's not in public.

It gives them an important feeling of seeing behind the scenes of tender intimacy.

What they don't like are what I call the beauty preservers. The hair nets, hair curlers, face treatments with creams at nights, etc.

Always blot off the surplus cream with face tissues before going to bed.

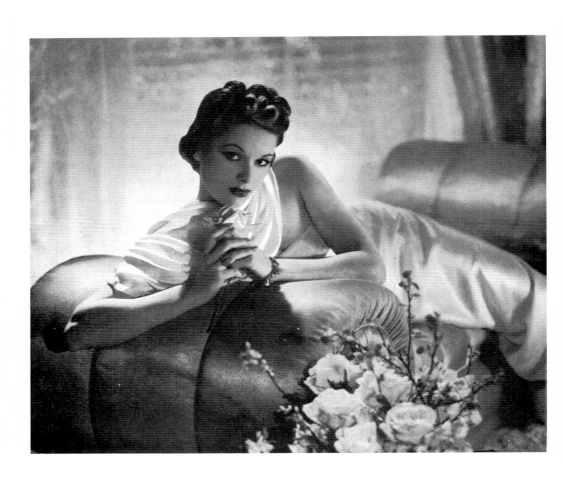

Tie your curls up with a pretty ribbon and leave the hair curlers for the time when he's safely out of the home.

And put the tiniest dab of perfume behind each ear.

Men are always foolishly sentimental about perfume—and the woman who wears it !

And keep an eye on your mind and outlook. Don't let either get stale or narrow.

Read as much as you can and have a hobby and some individual interests quite apart from your home and husband.

Many women when they marry seem to become colourless and lose their individuality. Don't let this happen to you.

BRING as much charm into your marriage as possible.

Be tender and true, sympathetic and understanding, happy and contented, proud of him and generous and make yourself always as beautiful and desirable as you can.

The more you do to make him happy, the more you forget yourself and think of him and what you can do for him, the happier your marriage will be and the happier you will be.

Keep the first tender sweetness of love alive, the wonderful planning together for the future, the tender little whispers in the dark together, the beauty of shared thoughts.

And remember that though you may have been married many years, he is still your lover ; you are still the one woman he chose for his mate.

Many women have a very wrong outlook on sex. They seem to think that having caught their man and borne his children that it is wrong to try and keep his interest alive.

They become almost prudish about sex.

They are absolutely wrong.

Sexual love is a lovely thing, a blessed thing. It is a thing of fire and passion and tenderness and mystery.

It is meant to be shared by each partner equally. No bigger insult can be given to one partner than the disinterest of the other.

How could it be wrong to try and keep this lovely thing alive between you ?

A man needs three things from a woman : companionship, love and tenderness. If you give him all three you need never fear the spectre of the other woman.

So if you can honestly say, when you have been married fifteen years, that you are still lovers in every sense of the word, it is something to be triumphantly proud of and humbly grateful for.

Don't be afraid to humble yourself. Humility in love is strength.

Remember the high, beautiful ideals of your marriage vows and don't tarnish those ideals by any act of unfaithfulness either in thought or deed.

For if you break your word, the promise you made before God, it will give you a secret feeling of shame. It will lower your self-respect, it will make self-approval impossible. It will put a barrier between you and your soul and the charm that lies within you.

And no fleeting happiness on earth is worth sacrificing that clear, honest joy of being at peace with your own conscience, for.

This lovely verse by Oliver Goldsmith expresses all the bitterness and poignancy of a woman who has betrayed herself by not being true to her conscience :—

"When lovely woman stoops to folly,
And finds too late that men betray,
What charm can soothe her melancholy ?
What art can wash her guilt away ?"

YOU may say : "That is all very well, but how do you find love ? I'm sure I could be tender and true as a wife, but I never seem to meet anyone who wants to marry me ?"

The answer is, you cannot find love, but you can help love to find you.

Stop seeking love and regarding each new man you meet as a possible husband. Men always sense this, and something in them, which wants to be free, immediately shies away.

Learn to express more and more the charm that is in you. As you learn to develop your personality, you will become much more attractive, much more full of charm.

And a woman with charm is always admired. Charm works like a magnet.

It draws people to you and, just as it drew your friends, so it will draw love.

Go about as much as possible, meet new people, make new friends, travel if you can.

Enjoy your life. Go through it with an air of expectation.

Believe that to-morrow love may come to you.

Have no doubts that you will recognize it when love comes. Your heart will tell you, the throb of your pulses will tell you, the shining light of your eyes will tell you.

For when a woman falls in love she enters into her kingdom.

THE ENEMIES OF CHARM

DON'T you feel a lovely new confidence already?
Confidence in yourself, in others and in the whole world?

Don't you feel more poised, more sure of yourself, nearer the fulfilment of all our dreams for you when we started together on this course?

For you are now a woman with charm.

You have untied the bonds that held charm captive inside your soul, you have set it free to light your life and the lives of all around you.

But there are times in every woman's life when it is more difficult to express charm than when her life is running smoothly.

Illness, periods, pregnancy and early motherhood are times when your bodily energy is a little below normal and it may seem difficult, too, to make the extra mental effort required to present the same charming "you" to the world as usual.

That is why I want to talk about each of these enemies of charm separately.

When you are ill, either slightly or very ill indeed, much the same rules apply.

Rule No. 1 is to keep yourself sweet and dainty all the time.

If you are well enough, wash your whole body over twice a day with a damp flannel and follow it by a rub down with fragrant toilet water.

If you are unable to do this yourself, get whoever is looking after you to do it for you.

Change your nightie every day and keep your curls brushed and combed and tied up with a pretty ribbon to match your nightie.

Keep a soft big baby shawl to cuddle into when you are alone and a pretty, fresh dressing jacket for visitors or when the doctor comes.

Keep the skin of your face nourished with face cream and your nails prettily manicured.

If you can't do them yourself, nurse will be only too pleased to do them for you.

Keep a tiny bottle of fresh eau de Cologne or lavender water by your bed to perfume your handky and dab a little behind your ears.

If you feel fragrantly sweet and know that you are looking pretty even though you are ill, you will subconsciously feel more at peace.

Keep everything near you tidy, the table by your bed and the bed itself.

Have a pretty vase of flowers to brighten the room and keep a lavender bag tucked under your pillows.

Now lie back on your pillows and relax. This is the most difficult thing of all about illness.

Not to worry about how people are managing without you, things you ought to be doing, when you'll be well, etc.

Put all these thoughts and worries firmly away from you. Relax completely.

A fretting, worrying patient is neither pleasant to look after nor to visit.

A charming, smiling, peaceful patient is a joy to care for and to visit.

Revel in the restful inactivity. Stretch your toes in your nice warm bed.

Stretch all over and yawn and you'll feel more relaxed at once. Practise the exercises I gave you for relaxation in Lesson 2.

Think about beautiful things, remember your beautiful memories and make beautiful plans for the future.

93

Try to think of this advantage of your sick bed. That it gives you time to pause in your life and think where you are going.

Time to take stock of yourself and make plans for the future.

So lie peacefully and dream and plan for your career, your home, your husband, your children, your clothes, your hobby, your interests, your games and your future behaviour.

When you are better, or if you are not very ill, make good use of this restful time to improve your mind.

Read the newspaper through from cover to cover each day—a thing you probably don't have time for in the ordinary way.

Read some of the latest books. Catch up with your correspondence, which you have neglected lately.

Make something beautiful with your hands, then you will not mind the body's inactivity too much.

Embroidery, sewing, knitting, crochet, drawing or painting—there are a dozen exciting things to do.

Convalescing need never be dull, unless you make it so.

Make this little vow to yourself when you are first ill :—

"I will try my utmost, not to be selfish or petty while I am ill and to make it easy and pleasant for others to care for me.

"I will not bewail my fate or allow others to do it for me. If I have visitors I will be cheerful and I won't discuss my ailments.

"I will follow all the advice of my doctors and nurses and not question it as I know it is for my own good.

"And I will not retard my recovery by doleful, self-pity. I will try to be constructive and hopeful in my thoughts."

⁂

PERIODS are trying times for any sensitive woman, especially as the changes that are taking place in her body have a certain effect on her psychologically.

I have talked with several famous doctors on how to lighten this distressing burden of women and I have learned many helpful things.

A woman often becomes more emotional, depressed, nervy and unsure of herself at these times.

The most important thing is peace and contentment.

For the first two days, do only what is absolutely necessary. Take a little more rest than usual and don't do quite as much running about.

Rhythmic exercise, such as walking or skipping or a rowing machine, is excellent, and is just what your inside needs, but don't do too much tiring running around, such as shopping or standing about.

Standing and slow walking are bad during periods, because they lead to congestion of blood in the uterus. But brisk walking or real exercise is good because it helps the circulation and avoids congestion. So either go all out or lie down. Don't moon about.

Try and take a short rest some time during the day with your feet up and your eyes closed. This will calm and soothe the nerves.

Warm baths are very good and help a lot. Try taking two a day all through your period. Besides making you feel fresher, they definitely ease pain.

Remember it is stupid and unnecessary to suffer pain at these times.

At the first sign of pain, take two or three aspirins with a glass of water at once.

They are harmless and stop pain in a few minutes.

If your periods are at all irregular or if the flow is abnormally small or large, do see a doctor.

I cannot stress this enough. Often it is some simple adjustment that is needed, which will save you future trouble.

If the pain is abnormally severe, see your doctor, too.

Remember that heat is marvellous for relieving pain. Curl up in a warm bed with a hot water bottle and you will soon feel fine.

Too large losses often cause anæmia, which must be counteracted as well as regulating the period.

If you are slightly anæmic, take Glaxo Fersolate tablets, three daily, for a week before the period, or liver with iron.

Don't let yourself get constipated before or during your periods as this often increases the pain.

Lead as peaceful a life as possible. Don't think of yourself as being ill. Just take a little extra care, such as not to get your feet wet, or over-tire yourself.

Try not to fret or worry about things and put off any important decisions or actions until your period is over as you have to remember that you may not be quite as clear-sighted then as usual.

Above all, don't let yourself be depressed or become self-pitying and be very careful not to pick quarrels with those around you.

The charming woman never lets this very personal problem reflect on those around her.

PREGNANCY is a time for happiness and dreams.

But it is also a time of occasional discomfort and a time when personal charm is often lost in thoughts for the new little life which is in the making.

Remember that there are two lives to be lived at once. If you neglect one, you are not being fair to your baby.

If you neglect the other you are not being true to yourself.

You've got to remain the same charming person to your family and friends as you were before this wonderful thing happened to you and, at the same time, lead a life of preparation.

With the added physical handicaps, some little mothers-to-be feel it is more than they can cope with and become discouraged.

Lead your ordinary life as far as possible and continue with your ordinary interests and hobbies.

But pay special attention to exercise, diet, rest and health.

For your baby's sake, lead as peaceful and happy a life as possible. Don't fret or worry or be angry.

Occupy your leisure doing beautiful things, thinking beautiful thoughts.

Just as the food you eat influences your baby's body, so the things you do and think influence his mind.

Never let your husband feel the effects of your having a baby. I mean this for your ultimate good.

If you are sweet and charming with him, a good companion, and still with other thoughts and interests beside the coming baby, he will be doubly grateful to you and proud of you.

Some women make their husbands' lives hell by their whinings and ailments and incessant talk about the baby.

Remember that though he will bear with you and sympathize, because of his love and pity for you, his admiration at your courage is a much greater thing to be thankful for and proud of.

Keep your person just as charming as before all the time. Your clothes, your hair, skin, body, and hands and feet.

Carry yourself proudly and easily and don't wear tight, constricting corsets. A comfortable corset, which gives you enough necessary support is better. There is nothing to be self-conscious about, so go about as usual and enjoy your life and everyone will love you for your charm and courage.

Though children bring a little bit of heaven with them when they come to a house, they also bring extra work and worry and ties.

A matron of a maternity home once said to me : "I tell every little mother when she leaves here with her baby in her arms :—

" 'Never let your baby be a nuisance to you. Let him fit into your household. Never try to fit your household to the baby.' "

She told me wisely that babies are adaptable little people and as long as they lead a routine, sensible existence, flourish, whereas husbands and families and maids are already set in their ways.

That I think, is marvellous advice, and it came from a woman who adored babies.

So if you are a young mother, remember that your baby should be an added blessing, but not your whole existence.

It is still important to live your own life and have your own interests and hobbies.

It is still important to keep yourself beautiful and charming, nicely dressed and well groomed.

It is still important to have friends and to be your husband's lovely wife.

Set aside special times each day for you and your baby to laugh, to play and to love one another. But remember that you have a life of your own to lead as well.

ENTERTAINING

ONE of the greatest tests of charm is when a woman can make the stranger feel at home.

Whenever you hear someone spoken of as a wonderful hostess you can be sure that it's not because she has a beautiful house or a priceless cook, but because she possesses this quality of welcoming charm.

The secret of being a good hostess is an important one.

It is a wonderful thing in a wife. Many men have reached high and important places in this world, because their wives had this charming quality of making their employers, their business acquaintances and their friends feel happy and at ease in their husband's house.

It is a thing born entirely from your attitude to others and from your interest in others. I can give you many practical hints on how to be a charming hostess, but the intangible something must come from you yourself.

The best way to develop it is this, I think :

When any stranger, friend or acquaintance or relative comes to your house, make them welcome in your thoughts as well as in your actions. Saying : "I'm so pleased you dropped in," and thinking "I wonder how long she's going to stay *this* time and I've got all that ironing to finish," at the same time completely disqualifies the welcoming spirit.

Take your guest into the kitchen or wherever you are working at the moment, find her a comfy chair and a cup of tea and then chat to

99

her while you get on with your work. And be glad that you have her to talk to while you work and let her know that you're glad.

Taking the guest into your home behind the scenes, letting her see and share in the running of your home is a subtle compliment, much more so than sitting stiffly talking to her in the sitting-room while all the time you're fretting to get back to your work.

THE Orientals have a charming sense of hospitality. Every stranger who enters their house is treated as an honoured guest. The best of everything is set before them and the whole family go out of their way to please them and make them feel at ease.

That is how it should be with you. No guest should be unimportant in your eyes. You should go out of your way to please and welcome everyone who crosses your threshold. Never be stiff or formal with anyone. Remember that even great men and women enjoy simple things.

Of course, hospitality is sometimes abused especially when the hostess is charming and always ready with a warm welcome.

Some people become a perfect pest, always dropping in and arriving at meal times or when you have other guests. If this happens to you, the best way is to be frank in your words so that there is no misunderstanding, but soften them as much as possible, with your most charming smile. Next time they arrive say: "Frank and I have invented a new rule for this household. We never seem to get an evening alone nowadays. So we're asking all our friends to let us know before coming round. We think it's time we had some quiet home life."

It is just as essential to keep an inner wall of reserve about your home as it is to keep an inner wall of reserve in yourself. That is the difference between a house and a hotel.

The hotel is open to all, to wander in and out at will.

The home is a personal sanctum to which visitors are invited when their presence or friendship is valued.

᪥

THE secret then of being a charming hostess is to welcome each guest in your own thoughts as well as your actions and to let him join in the household activities, not make any entirely new régime specially for his, or her, benefit.

Here are some practical hints which every thoughtful hostess should remember for her guest's comfort :—Among them are several ordinary rules of etiquette which you probably know already. But I give them to you because I think it is very important to *know* all the conventional rules of behaviour. When you are in doubt about whether you are doing the right thing, you cannot express charm. But when you know the accepted conventions, you can either follow them naturally or think up charming variations of your own.

1. A spare-room should be just as comfortable as your own bedroom with a bed you wouldn't mind sleeping in yourself.

2. Always tell your guest the times of meals and when the bathroom is free her first day, so that she fits in with the household.

3. Always see that all your guests know one another at a dinner or small party. Of course, at a large gathering this is impossible, so introduce late-comers to a little group of people.

4. In case you are in doubt about how to introduce people, always introduce a man to a woman. A younger woman is usually presented to an older woman and an unmarried woman to a married woman. In the case of two young people, at an informal occasion it is more friendly to dispense with the Mr., Mrs., or Miss, and use the Christian name instead. When you introduce two people, don't just say their names and then leave them

to it, feeling you've done your duty.   They will both be grateful
if you give them something in common to talk about before
leaving them.   If you know they are both interested in something, say : "You ought to have plenty to talk about as you
both like . . ." or "Miss Y has just got back from Switzerland."
Any little thing will do as long as it gives them a lifeline, to
start a conversation.

5. Never let your guests bore one another.   If you see a conversation
in the last throes of boredom, either break them up or introduce
someone new into the group.

6. If you give a party, make an unobtrusive little tour round the
room every so often to make sure no one is left out, or bored.
But don't worry people by inquiring if they have everything.
There's a great difference between a fussy hostess and a charming
one !

7. If you have guests staying with you, don't arrange something for
every minute of the day for them.   Most people like to have a
certain amount of time to themselves.

8. When inviting people to dinner or a party or even to stay, always
state the time you expect them to arrive and if it is for a visit,
state how many days you are inviting them to stay.   It is also
considerate to give them some idea of what plans you have made
so that they will know what clothes to bring.   In the case of a
dinner or a party always say whether it is evening dress or not.
This saves people a lot of doubt and possible embarrassment.

9. Devote one drawer in the spare room to all the little gadgets
which guests so often need and forget to bring or haven't room
for in their luggage.   Clothes brush, tooth brush, tooth paste,
hair brush, and comb, hair pins, curby grips, safety pins, needles
and cotton, scissors, notepaper, postcards, ink, a pen that writes,

bedroom slippers, and a spare nightie. It's great fun to be able to put someone up at a moment's notice and produce everything they need out of a magic drawer.

10. Make your guest feel honoured and pampered by little attentions to her comfort. Flowers in her room, bath salts ready for her bath, **tea** in the morning in a pretty cup, a bottle in her bed at night if it's cold and fruit by her bedside and a special case for her table napkin at table—they are all small gestures of charm.

11. Always have interesting books and magazines in your house for your guests to read. Keep a small, good selection in the spare room.

12. Never feel embarrassed because you cannot return the hospitality you receive. There is absolutely no obligation to do so. Entertain in whatever way is easiest and most pleasant for you. A tea-party or a sherry party can be just as much fun as the grandest dinner or dance. Whatever you choose always make your guests feel that it is fun to have them. Never let them suspect that they mean extra work or trouble and arrange things so that they mean as little extra work and trouble as possible.

The secret of being a good hostess is an important one. But the secret of being a good guest is an even more important one. You want to be popular, don't you ? You want people to love you and seek your company.

A charming guest is invited again and again.

The chief qualities of a charming guest are a holiday spirit, a sense of humour, consideration for one's host or hostess and the will to get on with one's fellow guests.

A charming guest arrives looking pleased and excited to have been invited, with a look of anticipation of fun to come. She joins wholeheartedly in anything her host or hostess suggests and she's always ready to see the funny side of things.   And she infects her fellow-guests with her gaiety and friendliness.

HERE are some practical hints on how to be considerate :

1. Always be punctual.   This is very important, as nothing is more annoying for a hostess than the lateness of her guests.

2. Never outstay your welcome.   If you're asked for a certain length of time, leave then.   Only stay on if your host and hostess are really pressing.   At a party never stay right till the end.   Leave when the bulk of the other guests leave.

3. Never forget to show your gratitude for hospitality.   The conventional bread-and-butter letter is such a cold, stilted acknowledgment, I always think.   A very charming way of saying "Thank you" is with flowers.   A tiny posy of flowers with a tiny note, "It was a lovely evening ; thank you so much !" is a gesture which will delight any hostess.

4. Always try to fit in with a household where you are staying.   Follow the ordinary routine, and make as little extra work and trouble as possible.

5. Help your hostess by helping to keep other guests amused and interested, and always be kind and sweet to everyone you meet in her house.

6. Don't expect to be amused every minute of the time.   Remember that your hostess probably has to attend to the ordinary running of her house.   Either offer to help her or be prepared to amuse yourself for a certain time each day.

7. Be ready to enjoy yourself, and let your hostess know that you are having a lovely time.

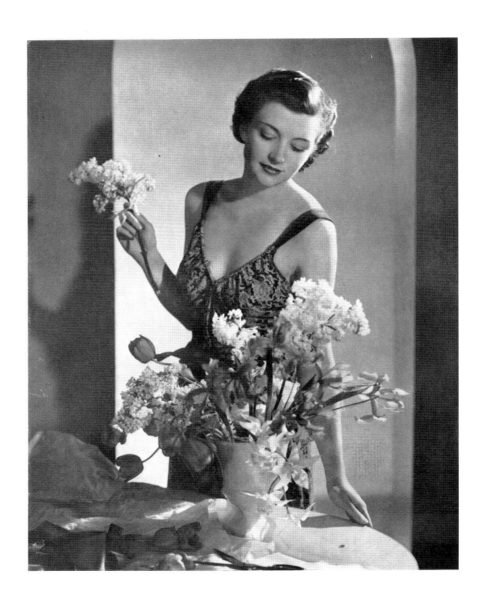

8. Never give your hostess' servants any extra work unless they volunteer to do some little thing for you. It is usually nice to give them some little appreciation of your gratitude when you leave. Give it to them yourself with an expression of thanks. It is much more charming than leaving it for them on the dressing-table. Never let the amount worry you. It is the gesture that matters. Give what you can afford, however small.

9. Be just as careful of other people's things as you would of your own—even more careful.

10. If you are invited to stay it is a charming gesture to take some little gift for your hostess. Flowers are always welcome, or, if she has children, perhaps a toy or chocolate.

11. Observe absolute loyalty to your hostess while under her roof, or when once you have accepted her hospitality. Never criticize her to others or allow others to criticize her to you. Never criticize your fellow guests while you are under her roof, either.

12. Try to be a "credit to your hostess" on all occasions. See that you arrive nicely and appropriately dressed for whatever occasion you are invited. If it is a visit, take the right clothes with you. If you are not sure what you will need, write to your hostess and consult her. Never let your hostess down by bad hehaviour or rudeness.

LETTERS should be charming gestures too. Every letter you write should have thought behind it.

Business letters should be dignified and gracious. Letters to your friends should express your charm and personality. Never write long, rambling letters because you think you should write a long letter. A short, sweet, amusing little letter is far more pleasant to read. Only write a long letter if you have something really interesting to say.

Choose an attractive, simple notepaper, and make it your own. Never use brightly-coloured paper or envelopes with gaudy linings. They are not charming. Express yourself simply, just as you would speak. Never be stilted or stiff in a letter. If you are doubtful about how to reply to a formal letter or invitation, refer to a book of etiquette.

Now here are two little exercises I want you to do to-night :

1. Think of the last time you had guests, and ask yourself if in any little way you failed to be a charming hostess.

2. Think of the last time you were a guest, and ask yourself if in any little way you failed to be a charming guest.

    Resolve to do better next time !

YOUR HOME

WHAT does your home tell the world about you?

Is it a perfect setting for your personality? Does it show that you are a tidy person, that you love beauty, that you understand the lovely use of colour?

Does it express Charm?

"Home" to you may mean just a tiny bed-sitting-room, but even this can be just as true an expression of your personality.

Your home should not be just a place where you eat and sleep and change your dress. It should be a setting for you.

A charming setting for a charming person.

LOOK round your home to-day, be it one room, two, three, or a large house
Study it impartially, as if it belonged to someone else, and ask yourself these
questions :

1. Does it look as if it had been planned with love and care, and not just a jumble of furniture?

2. If I were a stranger and entered this room, would I get a mental picture of the person who lived in it?

3. Is the colour scheme definite and artistic?

107

4. Is it overcrowded. Would it look more spacious with some of the furniture taken out ?

5. Has it got too many conflicting patterns, such as striped curtains and chair covers, with stripes of different kinds and colours, or a floral patterned carpet with floral covers and curtains ?

6. Are there too many nick-nacks round the room which give it a cluttered appearance ?

7. Does it look bare and unlived in, like a hotel room ?

8. Are there any dead flowers about, or vases in need of fresh water or badly arranged ?

9. Are the pictures suitable for the room, or have I hung them up just because I happened to have them ?

10. Does it look comfortable and welcoming ?

11. Are the lights arranged to the best advantage ?

12. Does it look bright and shining and well cared for ?

YOUR home has a big influence on your life. It is your own especial sanctum where you are alone with yourself or your loved ones.

Its atmosphere and appearance colour your outlook and moods, and to a great extent.

If a room is beautiful it becomes a pleasure to enter it, and your soul relaxes and revels in its charm.

To wake in the morning in a pretty room is pleasing, and this pleasure will reflect itself in your thoughts.

But if your room is ugly or untidy, or dirty and uncared for, it will give you a subconscious revulsion and an inner feeling of disgust, and this will colour your mood.

So you see it is important to make your surroundings as beautiful as you are able for your own good.

But it is also important to do so because of its effect on others.

A beautiful room draws you at once to its owner, just as you are faintly antagonized by an ugly, untidy room.

YOU may decide that your room is not all that could be desired, that there are many things you would like to do to it if you had the money, but as you haven't it'll have to stay as it is.

To turn an ugly room into a charming room costs remarkably little except in time and thought, and you'll find results will repay you a hundred times in pleasure.

First decide on your colour scheme. Remember anything you have already can easily be adapted to suit a new scheme by paint, distemper, or dyeing, so don't let that restrict you.

I have worked out many charming colour schemes for you to choose from to suit your colouring.

You will see I have worked out different schemes for rooms which face south or west and north or east, as the light and amount of sun make a great difference to the effect of the colours.

COLOUR SCHEMES
For the blonde with blue or grey eyes.

For a room which faces north or east, have the walls and ceilings colour-washed in a warm, glowing shade of golden yellow. Enamel the furniture in a deep turquoise-blue, and choose a warm, grey shade of carpet.

For the curtains and covers a patterned material of grey and turquoise-blue, and accessories in golden yellow.

For the blonde with brown or hazel eyes.

For a room which faces north or east, warm cream walls and ceiling, with jade-green enamelled furniture and a golden brown carpet of the same tone ; curtains and covers of cream and jade-green. Golden-brown accessories.

For the blonde with blue or grey eyes.

For a room which faces south or west, have the walls and ceiling colour-washed in a cool, pale shade of sky-blue. Enamel the furniture white, and have a primrose-yellow carpet.

Curtains and covers of white and primrose-yellow. Sky-blue accessories, slightly deeper than the walls.

For the blonde with brown or hazel eyes.

Choose a very pale shade of apple-green for the walls and ceiling for a room which faces south or west, and give the furniture primrose-yellow enamel.

Carpet in off-white, curtains and covers in off-white, and accessories in green slightly deeper than the walls.

For the brunette with blue or grey eyes.

For a room which faces north or east, have the walls and ceiling colour-washed in a warm shade of peach-pink, and the carpet a chocolate-brown colour. Enamel the furniture in cornflower-blue, with covers and curtains in cornflower-blue and chocolate-brown. Accessories in peach-pink.

For the brunette with brown or hazel eyes.

For a room which faces north or east, walls and ceiling in apricot, and furniture enamelled in turquoise-green. Golden-brown carpet and covers, curtains in turquoise-green. Accessories in a stronger shade of apricot.

For the brunette with blue or grey eyes.

For a room which faces south or west, colour-wash the walls and ceiling in broken white. Enamel the furniture in blue-mauve, and choose a cherry-red carpet. Curtains and covers in broken white and blue-mauve. Accessories in cherry-red.

For the brunette with brown or hazel eyes.

If your room faces south or west, choose ivory for the walls and ceiling, and enamel the furniture in apple-green. Curtains and covers in ivory and apple-green, with an Indian red carpet and accessories.

For the older woman with grey or white hair and blue or grey eyes.

For a room which faces north or east, colour-wash the walls and ceiling in a warm shade of rose-pink. Enamel the furniture in silver-grey, and choose a silver-grey carpet.

Curtains in blue and silver-grey and covers in rose-pink. Accessories in blue.

For the older woman with grey or white hair and brown or hazel eyes.

For a room which faces north or east choose a pale shade of lilac for the walls and ceiling, and elephant-grey for the carpet. Enamel the furniture in mauve. Covers in elephant-grey, and curtains mauve and a clear green. Accessories in clear green.

For the older woman with grey or white hair and blue or grey eyes.

For a room which faces south or west, powder-blue walls and ceiling, and furniture enamelled in a very pale shade of peach-pink. Carpet in French grey. Covers in French grey and peach-pink. Curtains in deep blue, and accessories in the same.

For the older woman with grey or white hair and brown or hazel eyes.

For a room which faces south or west, choose a silver-grey colour-wash for the walls and ceiling, and enamel the furniture oyster-pink. A deep rose carpet and covers of oyster-pink. Silver-grey curtains, and jade-green accessories.

For the red-head with blue or grey eyes.

For a room which faces north or east, choose a warm shade of beige for the walls, and enamel the furniture in turquoise-blue. Carpet of amber shade. Curtains in deep beige and turquoise-blue, covers in beige. Accessories in deep amber.

For the red-head with brown or hazel eyes.

For a room which faces north or east, have the walls and ceiling colour-washed in a golden-honey shade. Enamel the furniture in jade-green. Carpet of chocolate-brown. Curtains in petunia, covers in the same honey shade as the walls and chocolate-brown. Accessories in petunia.

For the red-head with blue or grey eyes.

For a room which faces south or west choose a cool shade of sky-blue for the walls and ceiling. Enamel the furniture in ivory, and choose a golden-red carpet. Curtains and covers in ivory and golden-red. Accessories in a bright sky-blue.

For the red-head with brown or hazel eyes.

For a room which faces south or west, choose ivory walls and ceiling, and turquoise-green enamelled furniture. Bronze carpet and covers, ivory and turquoise-green curtains. Accessories in gold.

IN the colour schemes I have mentioned nothing of materials or wall surfaces, as it is impossible to generalize. The type of person you are will determine the materials you choose ; something light and delicate for a fragile person, something rich and firm for a stronger personality.

If the room is small or dark a shiny surface is better for the walls and ceiling, as it reflects the light. But for a very large room a matt surface is really better.

WHEN you have decided on your scheme, have a grand clearance first. Get rid of any piece of furniture you loathe or don't use, and all the little nick-nacks which seem to accumulate, and never get thrown away.

Get as much feeling of space into your room as possible.

If your furniture is old or ugly, you can give it an entirely new life with a coat or two of coloured enamel. Walls and ceiling can be freshened and changed with colour wash or distemper and curtains, covers or carpets can be dyed at a small cost.

Don't overcrowd your room with pictures. Two or three in an average-sized room are ample.

Don't hang it up because it is a picture.

Study it as an essential part of the decoration first, and ask yourself these questions :—

Does it tone with the colouring of the room ?

Does its beauty inspire you ?

Do you hold it dear for some special reason?

If you do not answer 'Yes' to any of these questions, get rid of it or sell it.

Get something that does hold some meaning for you, or whose colouring tones with the room.

You can buy coloured reproductions of famous paintings very cheaply.

When you come to hang your pictures, make sure you hang them all at exactly the same height, and in the same manner.

In a high room the pictures should be hung much higher in proportion than in a low-ceilinged room.

Don't mix pictures and photographs in a room, as they do not go together.

And if you hang more than one picture do see that they have some bond of sympathy—of colour, subject, or style—between them.

Pictures are painted to bring beauty into the world or to give a message to those who see them. Some can see the beauty and message in one picture, others cannot, but can see it in another.

So choose only the pictures which please you, which hold something for you, whether it be beauty or a message.

KEEP your home just as fastidiously as you do your body.

Have a place for everything, and keep everything in its place.

Keep it warm and bright and shining, spotlessly clean, and its windows open to the fresh, sweet air.

Take a pride in the way you run your home, but don't let your home run you.

Some women become slaves to their homes. Fears that something will be damaged or marred spoil their enjoyment of it. Each person who enters it they eye suspiciously as someone who may defile the temp of their hands.

A home is, first and foremost, a place of joy. Somewhere where conventions are dropped, where one can relax and be at peace, or foolishly mad, as the spirit takes one. So never let the caring for your home spoil your enjoyment of it. After all, dirty footmarks and fingerprints can soon be removed, but nagging and cross words can't.

FLOWERS bring a wonderful charm to a room—and to its occupant.

Always try to have flowers in your room, even if it is only a single bloom.

Don't just dump them in a vase and then ignore them. Study them, love them, let their beauty bring you pleasure, and their fragrance bring you peace.

Never keep flowers one minute after they begin to wither, but make their lives as long as possible by cutting the ends of the stems before arranging them in the vase.

Flowers with wooded stems should have their stems split.

A good way to revive flowers that are flagging is to plunge them into a jug of water up to their necks, and leave them over night. This will give them a new lease of life.

Simple vases are far prettier and more flattering to the flowers than elaborate ones.

Learn to arrange flowers beautifully and to the best advantage.

Do not spoil the beauty of their shape and colour by arranging them with a mass of green foliage just to help to fill up the vase.

Green foliages, several different varieties mixed, make charming vases by themselves.

Remember that mixed garden flowers look better massed, and so do most little flowers, like violets, pansies and anemones.

Larger, more statuesque blooms, such as lilac, lilies, gladioli, are prettier not too crowded.

Flowers like plenty of water, so always keep vases filled up to the brim. Only change the water when it gets stale, as flowers don't like being disturbed.

Always set your flowers in a central position where they can be seen and enjoyed. A mirror makes a marvellous background.

Put them in your line of vision from your bed, so that your eyes drink in their beauty the moment you wake.

Keep a tiny bunch of scented flowers by your bedside to haunt you during the night with their delicate perfume.

Plants are lovely things to have around you. If you have no garden start a window-box or keep a single plant in a pot on your window-sill.

Watch the way it grows, the way it puts out fresh leaves, how its buds appear and swell until, at last, they burst triumphantly into flowers and turn their faces to the sun.

That is what is happening to the charm that is in you.

IF you run a house yourself, home will mean more to you than just a lovely setting.

It is up to you to make it a place of peace and relaxation for your husband, and happiness and fun for your children.

Work out an efficient time-table which leaves you time to romp with the children and the evenings free to spend with your husband.

Remember you are the pivot around which your little household revolves. You can bring charm into your house, or you can drive charm out into the cold.

It needs hard work and lots of it to run a real "home" for a husband and kiddies. It needs self-control, unselfishness, patience, understanding, and sacrifice. It needs a sense of humour, a young heart—and it needs charm.

But no woman is happier than she whose children dash home and boast to their friends about their wonderful mother, what fun she is, what a good sport.

And whose husband hurries home at nights, calls her name joyfully directly he enters the house, and folds her in his arms with a kiss, and "It's grand to be home !"

117

GO FORTH AND LIVE!

ND now the world is yours! Yours to enjoy, to understand, and to love.

Go forth, and live your life to the full. Go forth, and make the very most of the precious gift of life.

For you have learned the secret of successful living. You have learned the meaning of happiness.

You have discovered the secret of charm.

Poised, beautiful, sympathetic, intelligent, charming. Of you can it now be said:

"Heart on her lips, and soul within her eyes . . ."

We have come a long way together since we first made friends, and you became my pupil.

A long way on the road that leads to charm.

And we have reached our goal together at last, triumphantly.

Let us go over all the things that make for charm, the things that we have talked about together in each lesson.

Remember our first discovery—that charm was already there in your soul, only waiting to be liberated.

The necessity for being at peace with the world and with yourself before you could express the charm that was in you.

We spoke of your attitude to yourself and to others.

Of the importance of banishing self-consciousness, affectation, hate, pride, and nervousness from your life.

How you must honestly *approve* of yourself and live up to the highest and best that is in you.

The importance of keeping your conscience clear, and your mind untroubled.

❦

I SUGGESTED that you should read a beautiful poem each day.

Then we learned the importance of keeping yourself and everything around you fresh and dainty.

And we put something beautiful into your room to give you a feeling of pleasure every time you looked at it.

We determined to banish all that is ugly from you, and surround you with things you love and which please the eyes.

We talked together of serenity, and how to achieve it. Continue to practise the exercises I gave you whenever you begin to feel nervy, worried, or "tied up in knots".

❦

MAKE up your mind not to worry.

Count your blessings when you find yourself growing depressed.

Keep your eyes and ears open to beauty. Look for beauty in everything.

Meet antagonism with kindness—not condescension, but real, simple kindness.

You cannot afford to have enemies. Nobody can.

Never try to impose your will on another person.

Remember there is a lovely charm about a woman who doesn't take offence or gossip maliciously; who is naturally sweet-tempered.

Fill your mind with lovely thoughts and memories, and there will be no room for vicious, destructive thoughts.

Remember how we talked together on the importance of knowing yourself, and how we decided which was your theme type.

Remember our talk on dress ; how to use colours and materials to express your personality.

And how to be sure you are always suitably dressed for every occasion.

HOLD a pre-view with yourself and your mirror always before going out to make sure you are looking your charming best.

Freshness and daintiness always is an essential of true charm.

Feeling charming is half-way to *being* charming.

The charming woman never dithers in shops. She knows what she wants, and if it isn't there she goes to look for it elsewhere.

Be your age is a very important rule to remember when buying clothes.

Study other women of your same theme type, the way they dress, and the colour combinations they wear.

Don't be afraid to learn from others as long as it is right for you.

Use cosmetics to bring out every scrap of natural beauty in your face.

Cosmetics should never be used to hide, only to enhance what is already there.

It is up to each woman to make herself as physically beautiful as she is able.

LEARN to know and appreciate your body, and learn to preserve its flower-like beauty.

Keep your hair bright and shining, as it was intended to be, and find the right hairdressing for your face.

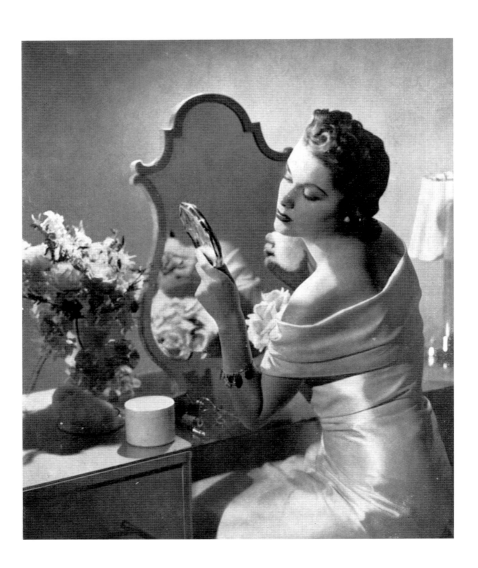

Keep your body in proper working order, for there is no greater enemy to beauty than ill-health.

Always be in love with someone or something. Whether it is love for a man, love for your children, your family, or the love of life itself, keep the love-light in your eyes.

It is the spirit of youth that you want to keep or recapture in your own movements.

Study things that are beautiful in movement.

Practise the circular wrist movement, trailing the hands after the wrists.

Practise in front of a mirror, doing all the little homely things you do each day.

Learn to love and appreciate your hands.

Practise walking beautifully.

Learn to stand beautifully.

Learn to sit gracefully.

Learn to run gracefully.

Keep your body young and elastic.

Check your weight regularly with the tables.

LEARN to be a good listener, but capable of good conversation if the occasion arises.

Not everyone can be a witty and amusing conversationalist, but every woman can have a fund of interesting and varied conversation.

Keep yourself well-informed about the world's affairs.

Cultivate a consecutive line of thought in your conversation.

Make sure you have no annoying conversational habits.

Make yourself as interesting a person as possible by reading and going about.

Make your voice as pleasing as possible to listen to.

Practise putting people at their ease.

Apply everything you have learned in your own home among your own family as well as to the outside world.

Learn to smile easily and expressively, and beautifully.

"Think" a little smile last thing at night. It will send you to sleep with your face relaxed, and a sweet expression playing round your mouth.

Make your laughter a pleasant thing to hear.

Cultivate a sense of humour, as it makes you wonderfully easy to live with, and endears you to your friends.

Never grouse if something is wrong or someone is imposing upon you. Say so frankly, and try to put it right, but don't grumble about it to others.

Never listen to other people's confidential grumbles. They are invariably just letting off steam to you, and will hate you afterwards for knowing those too intimate things about their life, their home and their friends.

Build up a little wall of reserve inside yourself, beyond which no one can go.

Discover the right perfume to express your personality.

LEARN how to make friends, and how to keep them.

Test your capacity for friendship and, if necessary, improve it.

Learn to express your personality and put it over.

Make yourself as interesting a person as you possibly can.

Keep an air of expectation of lovely, exciting things to come in your thoughts and on your face.

Always be kind and sweet to everybody you meet.

Never let yourself down by being rude or impatient.

As you become a happier, freer, fuller, more charming person, beware of becoming critical of others who have not learned to develop their inherent charm and personality in the same way.

Always be tolerant of others, and considerate of their feelings.

Cultivate a charming sense of tact.

Let people know that they can trust you.

Remember that the charm of being able to mind one's own business is a great one.

You can influence others far more easily by your own shining example than by trying to interfere.

One of the greatest tests of charm is when a woman can make a stranger feel at home.

A charming hostess is a wonderful thing in a wife. Many men have attained high and important places because of it.

Learn to be a charming hostess yourself.

Make every guest who comes to your house welcome in your thoughts as well as in your actions.

Never let people impose on your hospitality.

It is just as important to keep an inner wall of reserve about your home as it is in yourself.

Study my twelve practical hints for your guests' comfort.

It is essential to know the conventional rules so that your mind is at ease about whether you are doing the right thing.

LEARN to be a charming guest as well.

The chief qualities of a charming guest are a holiday spirit, a sense of humour, consideration for one's host or hostess, and the will to get on with one's fellow guests.

Study my twelve practical hints on how to be a considerate guest.

Learn to be a charming letter-writer.

Business letters should be dignified and gracious.

Letters to your friends should express your charm and personality.

Choose an attractive, simple notepaper, and make it your own.

Think of the last time you had guests, and ask yourself if in any way you failed to be a charming hostess.

Think of the last time you were a guest, and ask yourself if in any way you failed to be a charming guest.

Your home should be a charming setting for you.

Study it impartially, to see if you could improve it.

To turn an ugly room into a charming room costs remarkably little except in time and thought.

Choose your colour schemes according to your colouring, and whether your room faces north or east, south or west.

The type of person you are will determine the materials you choose for furnishings.

The size and light of a room will determine whether you have a shiny or matt wall.

Have a grand clearance before you start changing your room.

Get as much feeling of space into it as possible.

Learn how to choose and hang your pictures properly.

Take a pride in the way you run your home, but don't let your home run you.

Learn how to choose, arrange, and care for flowers.

If you run a house yourself it is up to you to make it a place of peace and relaxation for your husband, and happiness and fun for your children.

THERE are times in every woman's life when it is more difficult to express charm than when life is running smoothly—illness, periods, pregnancy, and early motherhood.

Learn how to keep charm in your life through these four rather trying times.

Love is the most beautiful thing in the world.

Every woman has the power to make some man happy and contented, and glad to be alive.

Find out through my questionnaire whether you are using that power rightly.

For a really happy marriage it is essential to face facts, and to be terribly honest with oneself.

Learn to breathe correctly.

Be interested in everything and everybody.

Never let friends or relatives be a cause of disagreement in your marriage.

You do not want to cheapen yourself by jealousy or bickering.

You must avoid all discord in your beautiful new life.

Never discuss your husband or your relationship with him with anyone, except, perhaps, a doctor or a priest, if you need advice.

Never let any little thing appear too much effort to keep your marriage bright and beautiful.

Don't let your mind get either stale or narrow when you are married.

Bring as much charm into your marriage as possible.

Be tender and true, sympathetic, and understanding, happy and contented, proud of your husband, and generous, and make yourself as beautiful and desirable as you can. Keep the first tender sweetness of love alive.

A man needs three things from a woman, companionship, love, and tenderness. If you give him all three you need never fear the spectre of the other woman.

Don't be afraid to humble yourself. Humility in love is strength.

Remember the high, beautiful ideals of your marriage vows, and don't tarnish those ideals by any act of unfaithfulness either in thought or deed.

You may not be married, and want to find love.

You cannot find love, but you can help love to find your

Stop seeking love and regarding each new man you meet as a possible husband.

Learn to express your personality and charm, and it will draw people to you like a magnet.

Go about as much as possible, meet new people, make new friends, travel if you can.

Enjoy your life. Go through it with an air of expectation. Believe that to-morrow love may come to you.

If there is any little discord between you and your loved one, make the first move to clear the air.

Read through the marriage service in your prayer book. It will explain all the deep meaning of love, and the beautiful mystery of marriage.

All these things make for charm. We have talked about all of them, and have pondered on them together ; how best to bring them into your life.

FOR I believe that Charm is one of the strongest things in the world.

A woman with charm is armed with a magic armour against all the hurtful, sordid things of the world.

It is not that she becomes smug or self-satisfied, but simply that she knows how to keep herself pure and untouched by the ugly things of life, and to look for beauty in everything.

AND now the time has come for us to say good-bye.

We must each go our own way now ; you to lead your shining new life, I to help others find the road to happiness.

If there is anything further you want to know ; something that puzzles you or is not quite clear ; or if you want to know how to use charm to solve your own problems, remember you can always write to me at the *Daily Mirror*, Fetter Lane, London, E.C.4.

We are friends now and I shall always be ready to help you.

But just before we part I want you to think forwards, to ask yourself where you are going.

It is easy in this busy, whirling life not to plan for the future at all, but just to allow yourself to be carried along from day to day.

But if you want to get the best out of life, to reach the highest places, to know the thrill of achieving your dreams and plans, you must pause in your life and look ahead.

Every two or three months have a little quiet session with yourself, and look forward into the future.

Ask yourself where you are going, where you want to go, and if you are going about it the right way to get there.

Ask yourself if you are content with your life as it is.

If not, and you long for other things, go out after them.   Things don't come to people who sit around wanting things and doing nothing about it.

AND so it is good-bye.

Go out into the world now, and spread the gospel of charm.   Be proud to be a woman, and do your best to make the name of woman stand for all the gentle, noble things it implies.

Live up to the highest and best that is in you.

Be true to yourself at all times, and never let that inner self down.

Be fine, and straight, and true ; hold your head up, and be glad to be alive.

Good-bye—and Good Luck !

Eileen Ascroft

EILEEN ASCROFT

Eileen Ascroft was born in 1914 in Reading. She wrote *The Magic Key to Charm* in 1938. The book is a collection of her hugely popular *Charm School* columns which ran in the *Daily Mirror* in the late 1930s. Although the book is a tutorial in the traditional feminine virtues, Ascroft was a pioneering female journalist who worked as a feature writer and columnist at the *Mirror*, set up the first women's page at the *Evening Standard* and went on to run a large magazine empire. She also learned to pilot a plane and was responsible for navigating a motor-cruiser on several cross-Channel expeditions. Her first husband was the celebrated film-maker, Alexander Mackendrick, and she met her second husband, Hugh Cudlipp, while she was working on the *Daily Mirror*.

Tragically, in 1962, Eileen Ascroft died of an overdose of sleeping pills

THE HISTORY OF VINTAGE

The famous American publisher Alfred A. Knopf (1892–1984) founded Vintage Books in the United States as a paperback home for the authors published by his company. Vintage was launched in the United Kingdom in 1990 and works independently from the American imprint although both are part of the international publishing group, Random House.

Vintage in the United Kingdom was initially created to publish paperback editions of books bought by the prestigious literary hardback imprints in the Random House Group such as Jonathan Cape, Chatto & Windus, Hutchinson and later William Heinemann, Secker & Warburg and The Harvill Press. There are many Booker and Nobel Prize-winning authors on the Vintage list and the imprint publishes a huge variety of fiction and non-fiction. Over the years Vintage has expanded and the list now includes both great authors of the past – who are published under the Vintage Classics imprint – as well as many of the most influential authors of the present.

For a full list of the books Vintage publishes, please visit our website
www.vintage-books.co.uk

For book details and other information about the classic authors
we publish, please visit the Vintage Classics website
www.vintage-classics.info

www.vintage-books.co.uk